THIRD EYE AWAKENING

A GUIDED MEDITATION MANUAL TO EXPAND MIND POWER, ENHANCE INTUITION, PSYCHIC ABILITIES, EMPATH, USING CHAKRA MEDITATION & SELF HEALING.

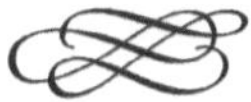

JOSEPH SORENSEN

CONTENTS

First, I will like to thank you for taking the first step of trusting me and deciding to purchase/read this life-transforming Book. Thanks for spending your time and resources on this material.

I can assure you of exact results if you will diligently follow the exact blueprint, I lay bare in the information manual you are currently reading. It has transformed lives, and I strongly believe it will equally transform your own life too.

All the information I presented in this Do It Yourself piece is easy to digest and practice.

INTRODUCTION

Did you know that your body is the home of certain energy centers that if developed properly can offer you the gift of spiritual vision? Do the words astral plane, aura, astral travel, meditation, and Third Eye mean anything to you? The truth is that many people are not familiar with the ideas and practices that have existed for thousands of years. For example, the oldest texts named the *Vedas* that were created between 1500 and 500 BC talk about the existence of the Third Eye, part of the chakra system, or energy centers found in the body.

Let us take a closer look at these energy centers. *Prana* or else energy is always flowing, as is indicated by the zero-point theory of Quantum mechanics, and particles never stay stagnant. Even when you are not moving, on a subatomic level, you are always moving. Within the human body, there are energy centers that are tasked to help it function properly. They function as a whirlwind of spinning energy that interacts with different neurological and physiological systems within our bodies.

Their help spans from regulating the organ function to emotions and even to the immune system. There are various chakras system counts but the most common one in western bibliography is the seven chakra system. They are placed throughout your body and start from the base of your spine to the crown of your head. Each chakra has its own frequency and is depicted through a certain color which specific functions that make us what we are: Human.

When we are born, each of us has a unique aura, a unique life signature in life. Your chakra system is part of that unique signature. As we grow, our chakras are able to absorb energy received from our experiences in life and everything that we learn. The way they absorb this knowledge is through reading your energy and take it into your system of self-understanding. When you go through difficult situations in your life, such as traumas, constant fights, and discouragements, your chakra system will react to these stimuli and block the flow of energy so as to prevent the flow of negative energy to your whole body. If they are not unblocked, this will result in the creation of a false identity that will hide who you truly are.

There are various chakra systems but the most known in the West is the seven chakra system. Those seven chakras along with their corresponding colors, and locations of each one:

- Root Chakra: Red - found at the base of the spine
- Sacral Chakra: Orange - found just below the navel
- Solar Plexus Chakra: Yellow - found at the stomach area
- Heart Chakra: Green - found at the center of the chest
- Throat Chakra: Blue - found at the base of the throat
- Third Eye Chakra: Indigo - found at the forehead between the eyes
- Crown Chakra: Violet - found at the top of the head

To some people, it may seem impossible that energy moves through the chakras or discs, but this belief has endured for thousands of years and there are many who have benefited from learning and taking care of their chakras. Yogis are one such example with another one being the *Ayurvedic* medicine where illness is viewed as the blockage of energy in one or more chakras. Acupuncture is also based on the practice of helping the energy flow through our bodies since blocked energy will lead to pain and disease.

Throughout the course of this book, we will analyze everything you need to know about the *Third Eye* as well as awakening it to gain all the benefits associated with it.

In the first chapter, we will introduce you to the world of the *Third Eye* because, in order to delve deeper into the different ways through which you will be able to awaken it, you need first to understand its nature.

In the second chapter, we will present you with the various benefits and dangers of awakening your Third Eye chakra, how to open your Third Eye s, as well as how to heal a blocked Third Eye.

In the third chapter, we will present you with the theories of the channels that make our life force flow throughout our bodies. More specifically, we will analyze the *nadis*, channels that connect the seven chakras and their health is extremely important in the awakening of the *Third Eye* chakra as well as the meridians found in traditional Chinese medicine.

In the fourth chapter, we will analyze the different planes of existence and more importantly their significance and how they impact us. We will discover the opportunities they offer us towards happiness and enlightenment, especially the astral plane. We will also guide you through the different methods through which you can enjoy the infinite peace and wisdom of this plane by connecting with it practicing astral projection.

In the fifth chapter, we will present to you with the various ways you can awaken and develop the gifts that have to do with your psychic abilities. Such abilities when combined with the awakening, development, and balancing of your *Third Eye* will give you the key to different worlds and infinite wisdom that you will be able to use to look out for both your own good and of others.

In the sixth chapter, we will analyze everything you need to know about auras such as how to see them, read them, and the meaning of the different aura colors.

In the final chapter, we will present you with all the benefits of meditation and analyze the scientific-based effect of healing or else mindfulness meditation.

WHAT IS THE THIRD EYE?

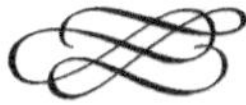

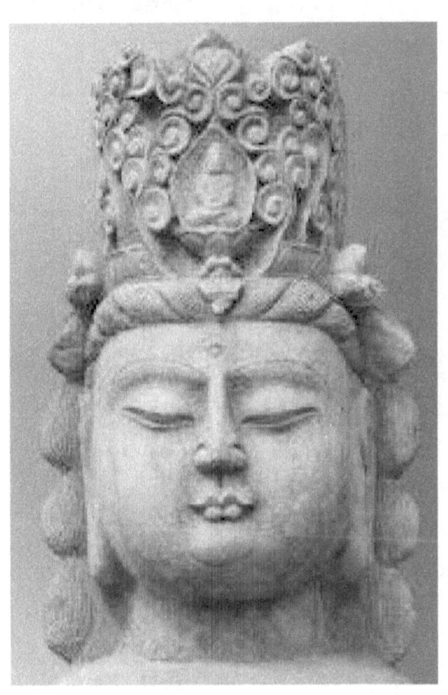

The *Third Eye*, which is also called the inner eye or the mind's eye, is an esoteric and mystical concept of an invisible eye located between your eyebrows on the forehead. It is the center of sight and intuition with its function being driven by the ideal of imagination and openness. In the seven chakra system, it is the sixth chakra and you may also come across the following names for it:

- Brow chakra.
- *Bhru Madhya.*
- *Ajna chakra.*
- *Dvidak Padma.*

The most common term in Sanskrit to describe the *Third Eye* chakra is *"Ajna"* which translates to "perceiving" and "command". This is the chakra that relates to the "supreme element," the element that combines all other elements in their pure form. According to yogic metaphysics, the sixth chakra is the center where the duality of the personal "I" is separated from the rest of the world and the personality exists independently from all else. In the words of Harish Johari at "Chakras: Energy Centers of Transformation".

In *Dharmic* spiritual traditions that come from India, the Third Eye is described as the gate that will lead you to inner spaces and realms of higher consciousness. In New Age spiritual tradition, the Third Eye is the symbol of the evocation of mental images with a deeply spiritual and psychological significance or a symbol for the state of enlightenment. For instance, the Third Eye is often associated with the ability to study auras and chakras, clairvoyance, religious visions, out of body experiences, and precognition. Those who claim to possess the ability to use their Third Eyes are most commonly known as seers. In Buddhism and Hinduism, the location of the Third Eye symbolizes the enlightenment that can be achieved through meditation.

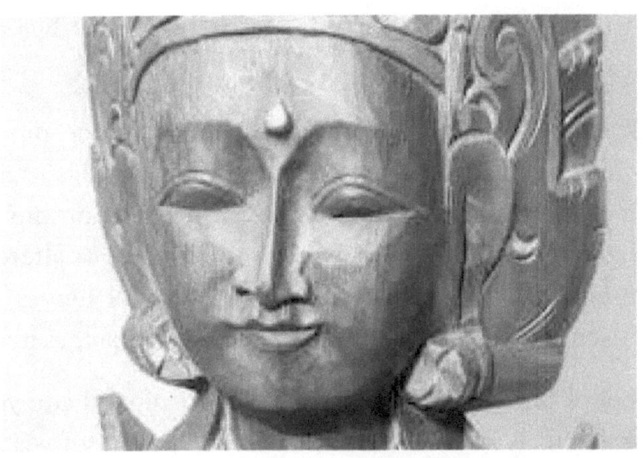

According to Taoism as well as various traditional religious Chinese sects such as Chan or Zen as is called in Japanese, the "Third Eye training" has to do with focusing all your attention to the point between your eyebrows when the eyes are closed and with your body positioned in various postures. The aim of this training is to get you in tune with the right vibration of the universe and build the foundation based on which you will achieve an advanced meditative state. According to Taoism which teaches that the Third Eye or the mind's eye is located between our two physical eyes and when it is opened, it expands to the middle of the forehead. In Taoism, the Third Eye is one of the main energy centers of the body and is found in the sixth Chakra.

The most commonly accepted color of the Third Eye chakra is the color bluish purple or purple. The Third Eye chakra is characterized by the luminous quality of its color and its soft radiance that reminds the one of the moonlight.

The most accepted location of the Third Eye chakra is between our eyebrows and more specifically above the bridge of the nose. Despite what most people think, it is not located at the center of the forehead but between our eyes at the center of the eyebrows. In several traditions, it can be located behind the eyes and in the middle of the head but you should keep in mind that secondary chakras reside in the middle of the forehead and for this reason, the Third Eye chakra is typically located at a lower level.

The sixth chakra is most commonly linked with the pineal gland which is in charge of wake time and sleep. This gland is found in the brain and at the center of attention due to its relationship with the effect of light and perception as well as the "mystical or altered states" of consciousness. It is located close to the optical nerves and as a result, it is sensitive to visual stimulations such as changes in lighting.

The symbol of the Third Eye chakra is very profound and yet simple in its meaning. It is ruled by *Krishna*, the Hindu deity of wisdom. The Third Eye chakra symbol is the Om in a position over an inverted triangle seated within a circle in between two lotus petals. If we examine them individually all these elements are representatives of wisdom. The Third Eye chakra is also associated with the element of ether and its symbol includes everything from meditation to prayer, the mantra of grounding, recognition of the Divine, and focus.

There is no animal linked to the Third Eye chakra due to the fact that may spiritual traditions and energy healers do not believe that the Third Eye is part of the physical body. The image created for the sixth chakra symbolizes two elements most commonly associated with wisdom the lotus flower and the upside-down triangle. As is the case with the throat and root chakra symbols, the sixth chakra symbol is linked with a dual purpose. Its geometric figure at the shape of a cone represents the channeling of information to the seed through which wisdom will blossom. If you view the triangle from another direction, the wide sides represent the growth of someone's wisdom that consequently leads to enlightenment.

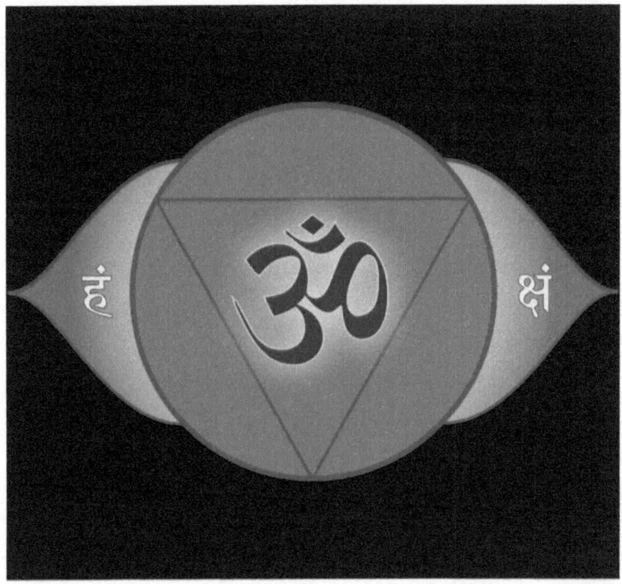

The lotus flower is almost accepted worldwide as the symbol of knowledge. Since it is associated with the Hindu deity of creation, *Brahma*, the lotus flower symbolizes:

- Fertility.
- Prosperity.
- Eternity.
- Beauty.

The mantra of "Om" is sacred and originates from Sanskrit which approximately translates to "the seed of all creation". It was chosen because its sound is what one may imagine the universal life force or hum of creation sound like. The sixth chakra is linked to the following behavioral and psychological characteristics:

- Intuition.
- Psychic abilities linked especially to clairaudience and clairvoyance.
- Vision.
- Perception of movements of energy and subtle dimensions.

- Illumination.
- Access to mystical states.
- Insight.
- Motivates creativity and inspiration.
- Connection to wisdom.

The sixth chakra works as a tool to understand the subtle qualities of reality. It reaches beyond our physical senses and in the realm of subtle energies. By awakening your Third Eye, you will be able to be open to an inner perception and intuitive sensibility. Due to the fact that it connects us with a completely different way of perceiving and seeing things, the images of the Third Eye chakra are hard to voice. The visions your Third Eye is showing you are commonly more subtle than any regular vision. They will most probably appear more vague, almost like dreams.

In order to sustain the awareness of your Third Eye chakra, you will have to focus on your ability to perceive things in a different way than you are used to. When you focus your mind as well as your consciousness, you will be able to see passed the illusions and distractions that stand before you and have the insight to create and live in alignment with our highest good. The sixth chakra is connected with the archetypical dimensions and the realm of spirits.

When your Third Eye chakra is blocked, you will become stagnant since you will lose your sense of direction in life. When this energy center is blocked you will, unfortunately, distrust your inner voice. The way you perceive life and the direction your life is headed will become a negative one and you will barely recognize yourself. You will be unable to let go of your past and you will be afraid of what the future holds which will make you extremely dogmatic about your daily routine, your beliefs, and the way you perceive others.

It is a fact that when your Third Eye chakra is blocked, it can gravely impact your physical well-being because it rules over your neurological function and your pituitary gland, the ability of your body to regulate sleep, fight off infections, and keep a balanced metabolic function will be compromised. In the end, you may find yourself suffering from insomnia, frequently sick, and develop high blood pressure. Some additional symptoms of a blockage in your Third Eye chakra are:

- Sinusitis.
- Sciatica.
- Migraines.
- Poor vision.
- Seizures.

In prolonged cases, there is a risk for serious conditions such as blindness and strokes. Some emotional symptoms of a Third Eye chakra imbalance are the following ones:

- Depression.
- Paranoia.
- Delusions.
- Anxiety.
- Nightmares.
- Vivid dreams.
- Heightened skepticism.

Added to the above, when your Third Eye chakra is overactive, it can cause disorientation and much psychic and psychological distress. The moment this energy center is set on overdrive, you will feel lost in endless phantasmagoric visions and overwhelmed by absurd pieces of information. In case you are not grounded enough, an overactive sixth chakra can sweep you off your feet. One of the most common signs of an overactive sixth chakra is an excess presence in a fantasy world which will make you lose touch with reality. Another symptom may be your being overly concerned about visions passing before your Third Eye. These signs can also happen when your sixth chakra is opening without the appropriate support and balance of the lower chakras.

On the other hand, when your Third Eye chakra is balanced, you will be able to see everything clearly. You will make decisions and function with a sense of neutrality. You will be concerned but not attached to one outcome of your decisions. You will be very focused, but you will be able to tell the difference between dreams and reality. An overactive Third Eye chakra will allow the constant flow of thoughts, something that can mentally exhaust you.

You will be intimidated when you have to make decisions that you would otherwise find simple. This indecisiveness will lead to clouded judgment, an inability to tell the difference between what is real and what is not, and a lack of focus. Some physical symptoms that will show you that your Third Eye chakra needs to be balanced are the following ones:

- Vision problems.
- Seizures.
- Nausea.
- Headaches.
- Sinus issues.
- Insomnia.

Some non-physical symptoms of an overactive Third Eye chakra are the following ones:

- Being judgmental.
- Metal fog.
- Hallucinations.
- Anxiety.
- Paranoia.
- Delusions.
- Feeling overwhelmed.

If you find yourself bombarded with visions that are too much to handle or filled with pieces of information that are coming too fast for you to endure and process appropriately, you can always make them slow down. Anchor yourself to your body and stay grounded as much as possible. The Third Eye does not physically exist but it is a spiritual existence. However, the senses received when the Third Eye awakens are physical. You will enter a new form of perception that will require care in order to be maintained and exploited to its most advantage.

Before we move on to the different ways you will be able to awaken your Third Eye, there is an important aspect you need to work on first: your sight, and we do not mean your physical one. Being able to see is one of the most important functions of people when it comes to conscience. It will allow you to discover hidden aspects of yourself. There are different levels of vision, but it would be wise to not bother yourself with lower astral clairvoyance and move straight to the vision of the self, which will help you eliminate the limits of your mind.

The different forms of vision have to do with the attachments of a person to pictures that travels into your consciousness. For you to attain the vision of self, you must be less concerned with your physical sight and pay more attention to its process. This will require your conscious state to expand. Once you achieve this, you will succeed in having a completely different perception of understanding life. However, do not underestimate the transformative value of vision by only believing it is simply a tool for perception.

One of the most common mistakes people make is to expect to see spiritual messages while relying on their physical vision and sight. This can't be done due to the fact that our mental consciousness is part of oneself, the blind part, so the first thing you need to do is leave your mind behind. Remember the phrase: "if you want to see, stop looking?" This is what has to actually happen to be able to see. There are several ways through which you can clear and open your vision such as practicing eye contact.

To practice eye contact, whether you are looking at your image on a mirror or at another person, you must keep a distance of approximately 3 feet. It is also advisable to have a blank background and to use candles, not electric lights. Also, keep in mind that if we look at the sun, our sight can be damaged quickly whether we have sunglasses on or not. So, you shouldn't gaze at the sun under any circumstance as well as you should not practice eye contact outside during the day so as to avoid any excess rays of sunlight that may affect the eye. The best set for this practice to be done correctly is in semi-darkness, indoors. To achieve a semi-darkness set it would be advisable to draw your curtains to make the room dim. Another thing you should keep in mind is to not look at the moon without blinking. It can also harm your eyes, but you can gaze at the stars with no fear. This is a practice that calms the soul.

Let us present you with a guided meditation practice that will help you be more aware of your sight.

- Sit with your back straight in front of a friend or a mirror.
- Close your eyes for about 5 minutes to reconnect.
- Open them and stare straight to the mirror.
- Stay still and turn your attention to your eyes and the eyebrows.
- Keep trying to stay motionless since it is not only the absence of movement.
- As you focus, you will realize that everything inside becomes still.
- The energy will feel as if it thickens and you will feel becoming denser.
- In this type of stillness, you achieved - connected stillness - is the one of the eye contact.
- With connected stillness, you will sense the energy of your eye connecting with your body's vibrations.
- Once this stillness reaches its climax, you will feel the need to move but you will not be able to. However, if the need becomes too much, you can move if this is what you truly want.

When you stare at something while your eyes are open, you notice all its different parts. Once you do this, you are able to process it in your mind and list almost its every detail. This is called the mental mode of vision and for you to be able to see auras and spiritual beings, you will have to turn this part of your vision off. Instead of listing the details of the things you see, you need to focus on the components of the object, you should be aware of the fact that you are seeing something. If you are not able to reach any type of awareness during the above exercise, stay still, and only be aware of the fact that you have an image in front of you. Then, forget about the image and start the exercise.

To complete the above practice of the eye contact, close your eyes, rub your hands, and put them on your eyes. Let them rest there for a few moments so as to have contact with your skin. You will feel the warmth moving from your palms, into your eyes. Stay this way for about a minute to enjoy this healing effect.

Another technique you can try that comes from hath-yoga is *trataka*. It has to do with having your gaze fixed on an object without blinking. You keep staring at the object until tears fall from your eyes because it is believed that this way all diseases are cured as the tears help in the release of many negative energies and poisons that have been resting for far too long in the eyes.

If you reach the stage where your eyes burn and tears roll from your face, it is said that you should be happy since various diseases that have been stopped and the tension in your eyes has been reduced. However, if you attempt this practice, you should not rush into it. Let yourself reach this stage gradually. As you practice, you will need less effort to stare at an object without blinking for a longer period of time. There will be times when your eyes will feel clouded, something that will make it unbearable not to blink.

Some common experiences you may have when you practice the eye contact are:

- The image in front of you becomes blurry and distorted.
- The reflection or person in front of you seems more distant than it actually is.

- The room seems darker and the colors of the room begin to change.
- You start seeing colors that are not there.
- The most common occurrence is you see another face in place of your friend's face or if you are practicing alone, your face changes and another takes its place. This happens because of:
- A spirit guide: it helps you achieve the ability to manifest your guides at will in a way that they can be seen by others. This way is one of the easiest for you to see spirit guides.
- A sub-personality.
- A past life: this may be the face of yourself or a person in a previous life.
- An entity: this presence is attached to you. It is often referred to as a non-physical parasite.

The best way for you to deal with such experiences is to not analyze everything that you see during your practice. It should be expected that various visions will make themselves apparent to you during this exercise and it may take you some time before you know what they actually mean. Write them down instead of worrying over them and place emphasis on the exercise and what on the contents of the visions you will encounter.

The Third Eye is not a visible actual Third Eye between our physical ones. It is more of a tunnel that starts from the area between our eyebrows and reaches the bone at the back of the head, the occipital bone. Inside this tunnel, several centers of energy exist that can connect you with different areas of consciousness. The Third Eye is the energy that belongs to the etheric part of the life force. This part of the body is connected to our physical body. The etheric body is the name given to a subtle or vital body found in esoteric philosophies which is the first or lowest layer in aura, terms we will discuss in later chapters. It is a fact that everyone has a Third Eye and can gain access to it. However, it is challenging at best and some may give up due to the work that needs to be done and its intensity. Let us explore the world of awakening our Third Eye.

AWAKENING OF THE THIRD EYE

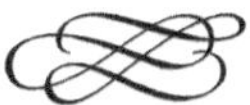

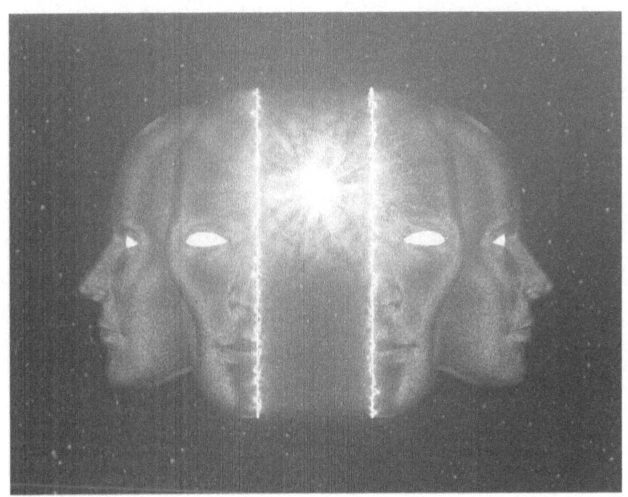

Have you ever had an intuition or most commonly known a gut feeling? This is the perception you draw from your Third Eye. For instance, have there been times where you just knew that you had to go to a specific place or contact a particular person despite the fact that you couldn't explain this feeling through common logic? The Third Eye is a unique organ that allows us to sense various things and it can be furthered developed with work. It can help you access intuitions that have to do with the path you follow in life, help you read the environment, and tune into the vibrations of others. In other words, awakening your Third Eye will not only enhance your perception but also help you connect with people who have a similar energy to yours.

There are many people all over the world, dedicating much time to awaken their Third Eye and then years to keep it from being blocked, overactive, or even closed. This is the case due to the amazing benefits of the Third Eye. For instance, achieving the metaphysical awakening of your Third Eye chakra will introduce you to a whole new world that you never knew about due to spiritual lethargy. This will allow you to understand the "Truth" that surrounds us by seeing the world as it actually is. You will have the need to live in a world filled with truth, love, and compassion. You will have the need to be free and see your connection with everything in nature as well as develop a strong bond with the universe.

You will harness the intuitive wisdom that resides within you, something that we all have the moment we are born. There are many traditional cultures that consider intuition the most important "sight" or "sense" that we possess and the various ways to open your Third Eye have, especially meditation, have been practiced for centuries. Your senses will become the right compass that will point you to the appropriate direction to be able to achieve what you are looking for. The term sixth sense comes from this concept. When you awaken your Third Eye, you will be able to instinctively read signals in a far easier way that will almost become like another one of your senses. You will feel as if you know what will transpire as well as the results of particular events. This is also why people believe that some of the most important prophets had succeeded in opening their Third Eye.

When you awaken your Third Eye, your Brow chakra will also be activated and achieve the alignment of your seven chakra system. This way, you will feel in harmony with the universe and energized. As a result, you will become a magnet for situations, events, and people by harnessing the power of love, gratitude, and positive intent. You will bring more beauty in your life and be more aware of the positive "coincidences" that will in turn increase greatly.

Added to the above, you will discover that you will sleep much better as well and your dreams will become more vivid since your pineal gland, the location of your Third Eye will regulate your sleep cycles. You may also experience lucid dreaming. In other words, you will be able to control your dreams and explore your true infinite self as well as the endless possibilities presented when we are sleeping. You will uncover the truth of the world of dreams being the same as the world in which we live. For example, you will see that the possibilities are unlimited and that we are in control of our own universe.

When you awaken your Third Eye and are connected to our level of existence, our soul will rise above our physical body and achieve astral travel through time and space. It is believed by many people that when we dream, what we actually do is astral travel and when our Third Eye is awakened, we will be able to astral travel consciously while awake, especially, when in a state of meditation.

Your imagination and creativity will also be enhanced since the pineal gland will be activated and as a result, you will be connected to the plane of existence that is the residence of our souls. In this plane of existence, there is only endless truth and love with everything that has already happened and will happen already existing in this plane of existence. After you connect to it, your creativity and imagination will be extremely charged. You will be able to find solutions to problems faster and more easily because the solutions to every problem that exists in our world, also exist in those higher planes of consciousness.

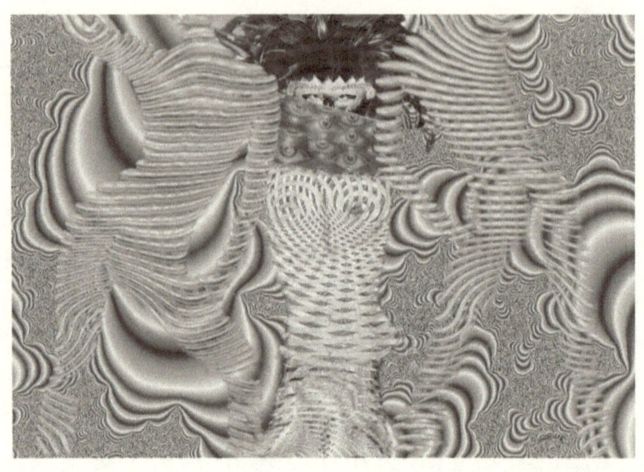

However, there are also several "dangers" of awakening your Third Eye with some of them being the other side of the benefits we listed above. For example, if you awaken your Third Eye at a time where you least expect it and you are unprepared, your sleep can be severely disturbed. More specifically, you will experience very intense nightmares and dreams that can frighten you a lot. This may result in waking up tired and having the images of your dreams returning constantly throughout the day and prevent you from relaxing as well as concentrating. This can be fixed by meditating before you go to sleep to help counter the side effects of such Third Eye experiences. This will also help your mind to enter into a balanced and calm state that will prevent the erratic input from your Third Eye. You could also keep dream journals since they can help you grasp the underlying themes of your nightmares and dreams and as a result, your Third Eye will stop overwhelming you with such intense images due to the fact that you will have processed the message or lesson presented during your sleep.

As we have mentioned, when your Third Eye first awakens, your intuition will intensify. Even though this is an amazing benefit for some, to others this may seem like more of a burden than a gift, especially at first. For instance, you may be extremely good at predicting how others feel or what is going to happen in your life but you may reach a place that it seems too daunting and you will actually feel unnerved by it and so find it less useful.

As time passes, you will improve the accuracy of your gut feeling and you can help this situation by not suppressing your gut feelings. Instead of trying to reduce the frequency of these feelings by ignoring them and pushing them away (which just makes them come back with greater intensity in the form of dreams), you should accept them. Try to remind yourself that such intuitions will be your guide to making good choices about yourself and others. Despite the fact that they may seem odd at first, they are actually the key to a more informed and happy future.

It is very common for people who have awakened their Third Eye chakra to report a sense of fearlessness, a sense that they are invincible, that nothing can touch them. The truth of the matter is that opening your Third Eye can be a very empowering experience and along with this empowerment comes an immense increase of self-confidence. The increase of self-confidence is certainly not a bad thing as long as it remains on healthy levels. So, what can you to keep this new fearlessness you will develop at healthy levels?

The first thing you need to understand is the fact that you have awaken your Third Eye will not make you omniscient. You will still need to carefully think about each of your choices in life before you act. Then, you will also have to engage in the rational parts of your brain to keep the balance with the immense intuition offered to you by the Third Eye. You will have to put some logic and sense into your intuition, especially at first. For instance, it can greatly help you to write the pros and the cons of a choice you are about to make as well as the intuitions and feelings that strike you for each choice.

Astral projection is another "danger" of awakening your Third Eye for many. As we established, with astral projection your soul leaves your body to travel somewhere else and this essentially happens while you sleep. This may be a frightening and confusing experience for some since as you get more spiritually powerful by awakening your Third Eye. This even can occur at unpredictable times which makes it more difficult to get used to. If you find yourself worrying over it, you should keep in mind that there is nothing dangerous about astral projection. You are not going to separate from your body, and nothing will harm your body during the time when you are temporarily detached from it. Try to understand that astral projection is a sign that your intuitive abilities are growing, and you become more in tune with the universe. As time passes, you will become more accustomed to such experiences to the point they will seem normal and even pleasurable as well as profound.

At first, awakening your Third Eye can be a scary and confusing experience leaving you asking how to close it since the new flood of information may leave you destabilized. There are some cases where you may find yourself wondering if there is a way for things to become the way they were before but it is essential to remember that you have just only gained access to information that has already been there. You will not be reading the thoughts of other people or change the future. You are only aligning yourself with cues you did not know how to interpret before. When you look at the big picture, the awaking of your Third Eye chakra can be much less frightening. Try to remind yourself that you are going through a spiritual awakening that can only benefit you in the long turn since it will make you understand the true purpose of your life.

Similar to being frightened, you may notice that you behave in inconsistent ways. This is a result of any major change that happens in life. You will need time to adjust to the new reality and give yourself time to train and understand how to connect your newly developed intuition with the way you behave. You have to be patient with yourself and not expect an immediate adjustment. Let the people you surround yourself with know that you are going through a period of adjustment and growth and let them offer you their compassion as well as support.

One last common "danger" is your Third Eye chakra becoming overactive. It may become oversensitive and have you experience some side effect such as:

- Vision problems.
- Seizures.
- Nausea.
- Headaches.
- Sinus issues.
- Insomnia.
- Being judgmental.
- Mental fog.
- Hallucinations.
- Anxiety.
- Paranoia.
- Delusions.
- Feeling overwhelmed.

An overactive Third Eye chakra will allow a constant flow of thoughts, something that can mentally exhaust you. You will be intimidated when you have to make decisions that you would otherwise find simple. This indecisiveness will lead to clouded judgment, an inability to tell the difference between what is real and what is not, and a lack of focus. If you find yourself bombarded with visions that are too much to handle or filled with pieces of information that are coming too fast for you to endure and process appropriately, you can always make them slow down. Anchor yourself to your body and stay grounded as much as possible.

The Third Eye can fall victim to imbalances by being overactive or blocked. When your Third Eye chakra does not suffer from not imbalance, it helps you see things in their true form, as they truly are but even the slightest imbalance can have a serious impact on your physical, psychological, and emotional health. Excess energy produced by the Third Eye chakra can send your mind into overdrive as if you have had too many cups of coffee. You will find it difficult to concentrate and even endure hallucinations.

The same thing almost happens when there is an energy deficiency in your Third Eye. You will find it difficult to process, remember, and concentrate on information. You will also find yourself being indecisive and be afraid of the unknown. There are many problems caused when the Third Eye chakra is imbalanced such as depression, insomnia, anxiety, and many more which makes it imperative for you to learn how it can be healed.

When a chakra is blocked, the quality, as well as the amount of energy that flows through the chakras, is very reduced. The goal of chakra healing is to support a balanced energy flow through our whole body or in certain parts of the body. The stimulation of our daily encounters, whether we talk about an emotional or direct physical stimulation, a little change happens electromagnetically in our body that is felt in our chakras. The quality and the direction of energy directed by each chakra changes, and the balance of the whole system fluctuates.

Chakra meditation is essential for healing and the awakening of the Third Eye chakra. There are several philosophical premises that support chakra healing depending on the healer and the tradition. There are, however, two most accepted theories. According to the first one, there are two essential flows of energies that impact the balances of the chakra system. A downward flow that comes from an all-encompassing and universal energy and an upward flow that comes from the magnetic field of earth and travels up to the chakras. These two main flows of energy are believed to bring balance to the whole system. There is another theory that stresses the importance of the upward flow of energy that starts from the root chakra and reaches up.

This dualism in the flow of energy reminds us of the philosophical subject "mind over matter" as well as the causes and the origins of the psyche. For the rest of the chapter, we will focus on the way energy moves through each chakra in order to bring balance and not pay too much attention to the philosophical foundation of the chakra theory.

In order to succeed in chakra healing meditation, you need to be relaxed and focused. The basis behind awakening your Third Eye chakra is to be able to see more clearly and within the physical realm and outside of it as well as awaken your intuition. Always remember that the Third Eye works together with the crown chakra so both need to be opened and balanced.

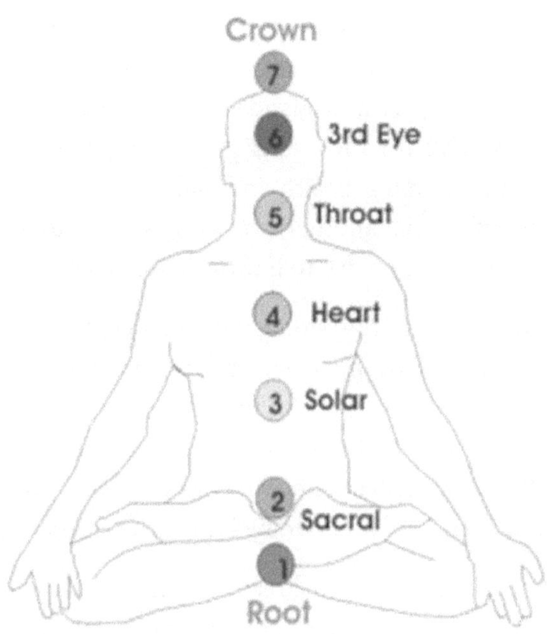

Chakra meditation is a set of relaxation exercises that focus on healing and bringing balance to your chakras as well as spiritual power to your body. There is no way that a person will be able to awaken his or her Third Eye as well as keep it open if any of the following chakras are blocked, overwhelmed or suffer from any kind of imbalance:

- Root Chakra: Color: Red - found at the base of the spine.
- Sacral Chakra: Color: Orange - found just below the navel.
- Solar Plexus Chakra: Color: Yellow - found in the stomach area.

- Heart Chakra: Color: Green - found at the center of the chest.
- Throat Chakra: Color: Blue - found at the base of the throat.
- Third Eye Chakra: Color: Indigo - found at the forehead between the eyes.
- Crown Chakra: Color: Violet - found at the top of the head.

Meditation is extremely important for someone who wishes to balance and heal their chakras. But how does chakra meditation works? The universe that surrounds us brings its divine energy to the earth and to our organs and glands found throughout the bloodstream and body. This life force energy is essential not only to maintain but gain our optimum health and wellbeing. As the chakras are connected and affect one another, working with meditation and this divine energy can help us work to our optimum level of balance.

To take your first steps in this wonderful practice that is chakra meditation, you should first sit in a place and in a position that makes you feel comfortable with your spine straight but not rigid. Then, focus on each part of your body that corresponds to the location of the seven chakras, starting at your feet and working your way up. Stay in each part up until each one feels relaxed by letting the stress melt away.

Next, you should focus on your breath. Do not force your breath but instead let it become deep and steady. As you feel your mind wander (since this is what happens especially to beginners), gently bring your focus back to your breath and keep your concentration fixed on each exhalation and inhalation you take. When you are completely focused, visualize the oxygen entering your lungs and then your bloodstream. See it nourish all your organs, cells, and muscles in your body and remove the toxins which are expelled with each breath you let go.

The next thing you will envision throughout your chakra meditation is the beating of your heart as well as the perfect way your body functions. You will see how all the parts of your body work together in total harmony. Your breath supports all parts of the body and all the parts together make your whole body. Your breath is the life force that flows and powers up the entire system of your body.

Then, the life that gives energy to your body is correlated with the air, the color of this energy will be a yellowish-orange color. This energy will encircle your whole body and enter your aura. As this energy enters your aura, you will see it become stronger and brighter, charged with tremendous energy. Do not forget to reach this place step by step. Keep your energy moving with each breath you take and let your aura become even brighter.

Now it is the time to energize each of your chakras starting with the location of the root chakra. Visualize a clockwise flow of energy as the energy in your breath feeds the swirl and gradually makes it brighter and stronger. This life force energizes and balances your root chakra.

Once your root chakra is prepared, it is time to move up to the sacral chakra. The same process should be followed here too, as well as with the solar plexus chakra, the heart chakra, the throat chakra, the Third Eye chakra, and in the end the crown chakra. Each will be infused with energy to bring balance. Do not worry about the time you should stay at each location. Spend as much time as needed to feel each part of your body that corresponds to its respective chakra cleansed, energized, and stress-free.

Do not skip a chakra because they are connected and influence each other. So, you should start from the bottom and work up, energizing each chakra before you move on because the whole process will have an adverse effect. The last step in chakra meditation is to envision all your chakras (once they are fully energized as well as your aura) becoming clearer, brighter, and extremely charged from this life energy.

In the end, you can open your eyes and stay in position to relax for a few minutes while keeping your eyes open. Take care to pay attention to your newly energized body and how amazing it feels. It is important to work as much as you can on this meditation and pay attention to all of your chakras since they are one connected system. You can't focus on one part of the system and hope the problem is fixed, you need to meditate on all of them for the system to be balanced.

As you gain more experience, you will be better at detecting individual blockages and able to direct your meditation to focus on specific chakras. You should also keep in mind that to practice this, you may need approximately an hour and maybe a little more. So, if you are in a hurry choose the appropriate time because each chakra alone needs several minutes to be properly treated and energized.

Besides chakra meditation, there are several other ways for you to bring the balance once more to your Third Eye such as sound therapy, acupressure, Reiki, and acupuncture. Essential oils can also help in the healing of the Third Eye. You can pour some drops on the forehead and more specifically at the location of the Third Eye chakra. The most helpful ones are the following:

- Frankincense.
- Marjoram.
- Clary Sage.
- Juniper.
- Sandalwood.
- Rosemary.

There are also several healing foods that can help you heal and maintain a balanced Third Eye chakra and those foods have as their main theme the color purple. Dark blue or purple foods can enhance the functions of the sixth chakra.

- Blueberries.
- Eggplant.
- Purple cabbage.
- Purple kale.
- Purple peppers.
- Plums.

The Third Eye chakra rules what is most commonly referred to as the sixth sense. There are numerous healing stones that work perfectly with the sixth chakra and these are listed below:

- Amethyst: It is used to balance, open, and stimulate. It is a healing stone that gives us healing, wisdom, and protects us from harm.
- Purple Fluorite: It is used to balance and stimulate. This is the stone that dispels negativity and promotes focus, mental clarity, and intuition.
- Moldavite: It is used to balance, stimulate, and to cleanse. It can clear negativity and restore balance to the whole chakra system. It also enhances dream recall and dreams in general.
- Black Obsidian: It is used to balance and stimulate. It is great for chakra blockages by expelling negativity and helping you enhance your emotional control.

The above chakra healing stones are perfect to use when you experience signs of fatigue, emotional issues, inability to focus, and headaches. When compared along with meditation, a good diet, and yoga, these crystals can help you balance your Third Eye perfectly.

The cultivation of silence in your mind through meditation or by simply enjoying the calm in nature will also greatly help when trying to heal your Third Eye. This happens because the perception of the Third Eye will elevate your senses to more subtle levels that some call psychic abilities or the realm of the invisible. You will be able to hear information and messages that stem from your Third Eye, but you have to be ready to receive the whispers of its wisdom. Your mind should not be busy with anything else or you will certainly miss all that it has to say.

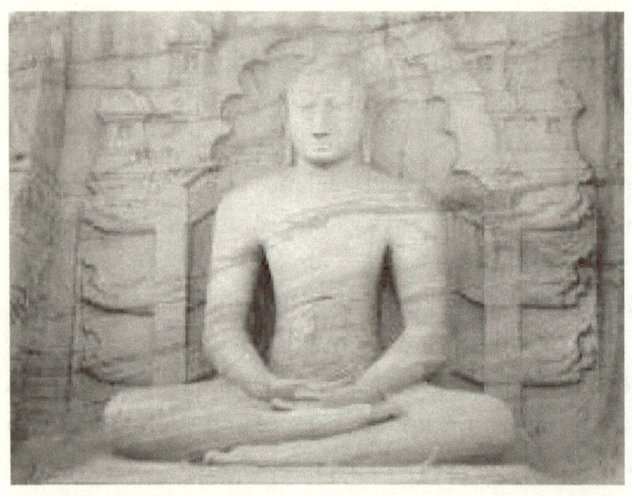

In order to be able to awaken your Third Eye, meditation is essential. As is the case with any type of meditation, Third Eye meditation needs you to remain in a calm and soothing environment to benefit from is calming vibes and sounds. Let us see the steps of a Third Eye chakra meditation that will help you in awakening it.

- To start with, sit in a comfortable position on the floor or in a chair. Keep your spine straight with your shoulders relaxed and your hands on the knees.
- Your stomach, face, and jaw must be completely opened and relaxed to the positive inflow of energy.
- When these are achieved, bring together the thumb and the index finger and gently close your eyes.
- Breathe slowly by exhaling and inhaling through your nose.
- While keeping your eyes closed try to look up to your Third Eye that is found between your eyebrows.
- You can also use your fingers to pinpoint the location.
- Then, breathe slowly and concentrate on this point.
- Keep doing so until you find a bluish-white or white light surrounding you.
- As you do this, you will enter a transcendental form of healing with your concentration being at its most effective and at its peak.

- This state is the one you achieve when you let go of bad thoughts, energies, or only focus on enhancing the abilities of your Third Eye chakra.
- Focus should be your top priority.
- Stay in this position for about 10 to 20 minutes.
- You can use relaxing music to aid in the channeling of your concentration powers.
- End the third chakra meditation session by exhaling a deep breath.
- Bring your palms together and place them in front of your heart and return them to the initial position.
- Blink your eyes and remain to this position for about two seconds before moving on with your day.
- Practice this Third Eye chakra meditation every day in the morning or before you go to bed and you will see the powers of your Third Eye growing little by little.

Cultivating and sharpening your intuition will also help you both awaken and heal your Third Eye. Since it is the center of higher wisdom, vision, and insight, you need to get in touch with the meaning of your dreams or get to know how to read tarot cards and a horoscope. You need to find daily activities that will sharpen your intuition because the sixth chakra rests at one of the main higher levels of intuition and perception. Be curious and learn such techniques. It may take time, but you will familiarize yourself with these practices and gain more confidence in your abilities.

Creativity is also essential for the Third Eye, so you should nurture it and let it flow freely. Let your imagination loose by starting a new craft or art. Do not aim for perfection but to let your inspiration flow without stopping it and be prepared to be surprised by the results. Creativity will loosen your rational mind that tends to control everything. When this part of your mind is calmed and you get the reigns of how reality should be, this will open up many possibilities and your Third Eye will have the space to develop and fully unfold.

For you to balance and awaken the abilities of your Third Eye, you need first to learn how to stand on both of your feet, you need to ground yourself. This way, you will have the foundations that will allow you to interpret your perceptions with confidence and clarity. You need to gain enough energy to flow through your whole body and energize your whole chakra system to support the health of this channel of perception. When you are grounded, you will have enough energy to expand your mind to more subtle dimensions of perception and receive as well as accept information that may seem unusual, disturbing, or unfamiliar to the common mind.

Grounding meditation can be extremely beneficial for awakening your Third Eye. With grounding meditation, you will enhance the physical connection between the electrical frequencies of the Earth and the human body. When you practice grounded meditation, you will be able to focus your mind on the present moment as well as be more aware and balanced. There are many times that our minds become unfocused to the extent that it makes you feel uneasy, uncomfortable, and restless. When you ground yourself you will feel centered, peaceful, and calm.

Some of the benefits of grounded meditation include:

- Increased mental clarity.
- Increased emotional clarity.
- Stress reduction.
- Enhanced feeling of calm.
- Enhanced feelings of peacefulness.
- Improved health.
- Increased energetic awareness.

Before you start your meditation practice, you should try to connect with the physical environment around you as well as the spiritual energy of everything that surrounds you. Through grounding with the energy of the Earth, you will be more aware of the energy your body has. For instance, you can walk barefoot on grass or wet sand and feel the earth under your feet. Keep your focus on the earth underneath your feet. Make contact with a tree, a flower, or any other living organism from Earth to connect with nature. Then follow the steps presented below:

- Turn off all electronic devices.
- Find a quiet place where no one will disturb you for about 20 minutes and if possible, it should be outside where you can rest your bare feet on the soil or the grass.
- If you can't be outside, you can use an Earthing Band or an Earthing Mat to connect yourself with the energy of the Earth.
- Sit on the ground or in a chair and place your feet on the ground.
- Close your eyes and place your hands on your lap with your palms facing upward.
- Stay in this position for a few seconds to make sure your body is comfortable.
- Then, visualize yourself resting against a tree trunk.
- Focus on the energy that resides in your body and how it flows downward to the earth.
- The tree is the extension of your body that extends through your feet.
- Keep imagining this tree trunk that travels through the Earth until it reaches the center of the Earth.
- As you are breathing, let all the negative feelings you may have leave your body.
- Any feelings of anger, bitterness, pain, and frustration will vanish from inside you.
- Then, push your energy upwards and imagine the energy of the Earth flowing back through your trunk.

You can also do the following:

- Visualize a breathtaking mountain.
- Picture its details and its stable presence as it stays grounded in the Earth.
- Then, lead the mountain inside yourself.

- Imagine yourself becoming the mountain.
- Visualize yourself sitting in calm and stillness by only observing and resting as the various weather types of seasons and storms pass you by.
- Feel yourself staying rooted still while in the middle of continuous change of external and internal experience.

To finish your meditation session:

- Before you open your eyes, revel in the emotions of calm and centeredness for a while.
- When you are ready, bring your mind back to your body.
- Then, open your eyes.
- Whenever you feel unfocused, shut your eyes and visualize the connection you have already shared with the Earth.

As you practice grounding meditation more and more, the whole process will be more automatic. A few moments a day for practice will be very beneficial since you will have a better energy and focus on yourself as well as find inner peace and calmness no matter where you are. Meditation is key to awakening your Third Eye and grounding meditation is an essential practice for this purpose.

Mindful breathing can also help you calm your mind and awaken, as well as cleanse, the Third Eye. Mindfulness is the ability to stay fully present, bringing your focus to your experiences as they happen in the present. Adding the color indigo to your life, a combination of violet and blue can help in healing the Third Eye chakra since that is its color. Introduce purple and blue hues to your office and home and surround yourself with this calming color that can boost the flow of energy and heal the Third Eye.

When practicing Third Eye meditation, it is best to do so after having woken up recently from a state of sleep. So, it would be best to do so after an afternoon nap or in the morning. This is true because after sleeping your brain already is in a state similar to meditation, in other words, in a very relaxed state with enhanced intuition and inner awareness with low anxiety and stress levels. In such a case, you can also try this Third Eye awakening meditation:

- Dedicate at least 30 minutes for Third Eye meditation.
- Turn off all electronic devices to avoid any distractions.
- Make sure that your clothes feel comfortable.
- Sit on the ground in the lotus position as shown below, to make sure that all your chakras are aligned.

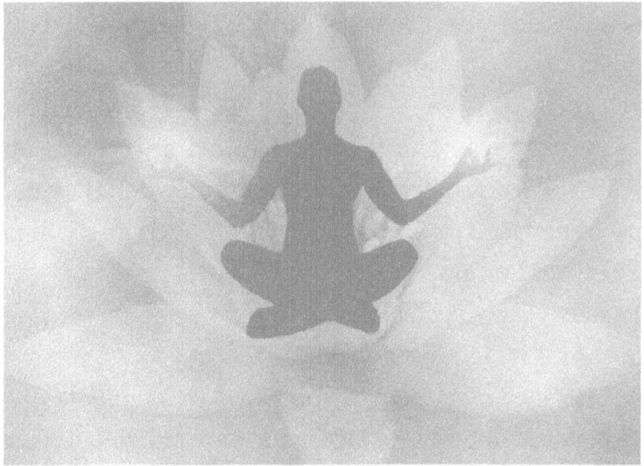

- If you are not comfortable to stay in this position, you can lie down.
- Start relaxing all the muscles of your body, beginning with your toes and work your way up to the head.
- Visualize each ligament, bone, and muscle relaxing.
- Breathe calmly and be mindful of your breath.
- Then, visualize a wave of calm energy that surrounds your body.
- Focus on its warmth as it reaches higher parts of your body.
- Draw this energy gently and solely to the center of your head, located between your eyebrows.
- Don't try to think or process any image. Simply let go of all aversion and attachments as if nothing matters.

- Focus on how it feels as your body becomes lighter and gravity fades away.
- Focus on your breath and imagine a white ball of light spinning 360 degrees at the center of your mind.
- Pay attention as this ball expands and accept its presence.
- As it expands, let it stream out through the center of your forehead.
- Let go of any thoughts, letting them come and go.
- Keep this light open and see what it presents you with, be it colors, pictures, or information.
- If you wish to connect with a spirit guide or mother nature, this is the time to do so. You can call them internally or vocally.
- Keep repeating your words like a mantra until they respond to you. You will know how they will respond when they do.
- Do not be alarmed or afraid when they do because you may break the meditation.
- You can also ask your Third Eye to send you a message for insight or information.
- This experience may seem to you like a dream but as you practice, you will be able to manifest and cultivate higher knowledge into your physical existence.

Keep in mind that Third Eye meditation is an ability that can take years to master and for this reason, most people go no further than only sitting down to meditate. To make things easier, you should first start with basic meditation such as grounding meditation because the development of a centered, present, and balanced state is extremely important for you to open your Third Eye.

Trust your experiences and have faith in them. There is no point worrying over things when you can let your experiences guide you. As time passes and you practice more, your Third Eye and your abilities connected to it will flourish. You will grow in precision and reliability. Keep in mind that you should not analyze anything during an experience you have or you will lose your perception immediately.

Practice your stillness and do not react when something happens. Once your experience is over completely, you can start analyzing it as much as you wish. However, you should always remember that you will not always be benefited by analyzing each of your experiences.

Meditating is not a boring experience; it is something you can enjoy and have fun with. Even though you should adhere to the techniques strictly, this does not mean that you should not experiment and have fun with meditation now and then. Always remember that you will be able to see the world from different perspectives since you will gain access to knowledge that people who have not yet awoken their Third Eye are ignorant about.

Despite the fact that awakening your Third Eye needs time, do not give up and practice as much as you can. Meditate all the time to reap all the benefits associated with developing your Third Eye. There is no need to delay your decision to start practicing. Even if you think that 20 minutes to half an hour is time you don't have, start small and work your way up. It is a self-transformative experience and it is a waste of time to delay finding your purpose in life.

CHANNEL RELEASE

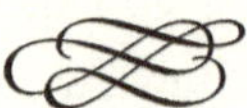

According to Hinduism, the Three Bodies Doctrine maintains that the human body consists of three bodies *sariras* coming from *Brahman* by *avidya*. *Brahman* in Hinduism is the highest Universal Principle, in other words, the Ultimate Reality in our Universe. In the most prominent schools of Hindu philosophy, it is the formal, material, efficient, and final cause of everything that exists. It is the eternal and infinite truth which never changes and yet is the one that causes everything change that happens.

Brahman is the one binding unity that brings together everything different in the universe. It is an essential concept in the *Vedas* and for this reason, it is discussed extensively in the early *Upanishads*, which are ancient Sanskrit texts part of the *Vedas* talking about the ideas and spiritual teaching of Hinduism. The *Vedas* view *Brahman* as the Cosmic Principle. The Three Bodies Doctrine is inherently related to the seven chakras and by extension to the Third Eye.

Avidya, which along with *Brahman* creates the three bodies is the Sanskrit word that can be translated as misconception, incorrect knowledge, ignorance, and misunderstanding as opposed to *Vidya*. You can find it being used extensively in Hindu texts such as the

Upanishads and various other Indian religions such as *Jainism* and *Buddhism* in the context of metaphysics.

In every Dharmic system, *Avidya* is the one that shows the fundamental misperception and ignorance of the phenomenal world. On the other hand, the various religions of India do not agree on the details. For instance, Hinduism considers as a form of *Avidya* the misconceptions and denial of *Atman* – self, soul. According to Buddhism, a form of *Avidya* is the misconceptions and denial of the *An-atman* – non-self, non-soul.

The three bodies are often correlated with the five koshas or sheaths that cover the *atman* – the soul. *Sthula sarira* is the gross body, our physical, material mortal body that acts through breathing, moving, and eating. It is built by different components that are created by a person's karmas or else actions, in their past life. The main features of this body are:

- *Sambhava* or birth,
- *Jara* or old age – ageing.
- *Maranam* or death.
- The "Waking State"

Sukshma *sarira* is our subtle body is the body of the mind and its essential energies that work to keep our physical body alive. Along with the casual body, they are the *jiva* or transmigrating soul that separates from the gross body when we perish. The subtle body is the home of the chakras and by extension the Third Eye, which are connected by channels named *nadis*, a term we are going to analyze shortly. This body is made up from the following five subtle elements:

- *Vagadipanchakam*: the five organs of action – hands, speech, legs, genitals, and anus.
- *Sravanadipanchakam*: the five organs of perceptions – ears, tongue, eyes, skin, and nose.
- *Pranapanchakam*: the five-fold essential breath – *Apana* or the expelling of waste from the body, *Prana* or respiration, *Vyana*

or blood circulation, *Samana* or digestion, *Udana* or else actions such as crying, sneezing, vomiting.

- *Buddhi*: the discriminating wisdom, the Intellect
- *Manas*: the mind

Karana Sarira is the casual body and refers to the highest body that covers our true soul. It is the cause of the gross and subtle body and its function is restricted to be the seed of the gross and subtle body. Its origins can be traced in *avidya* or ignorance of the true identity of the *atman*. According to *Swami Sivananda*, a Hindu spiritual teacher, the causal body as "The beginningless ignorance that is indescribable". The casual body is essentially characterized by ignorance, emptiness, and darkness.

The three bodies doctrine is essential in the chakra concept because the purification of the chakra and will lead to the purification of all the bodies and then, they will become one, they will become harmonious. This will lead you to be more energetic, full-hearted, and strong. If your goal is to grow spiritually, you need to remove any impurities from all of the three bodies in order to discover your true self and achieve your peace of mind and good health.

Nadi is the Sanskrit word for pipe, blood vessel, tube, nerve, and pulse. It is a term that describes the channels through which the energies – *prana* - of the physical, the casual, and the subtle body flow. The *nadis* are the ones to connect the chakras. There are three main *nadis* that go from the base of the spine and to the head:

- The *Ida* on the left side of the spine – left channel.
- The Sushumna runs through the seven chakras and along the spinal cord in the center – central channel.
- The *Pingala* on the right side of the spine – right channel.

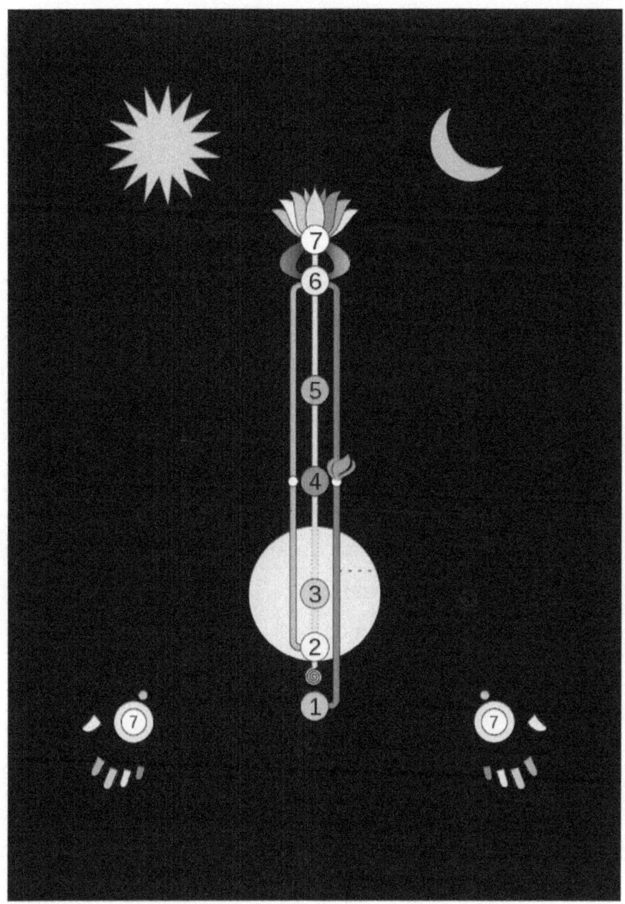

In Hindu philosophy, *nadi* is an essential concept mentioned various times in texts 3,000 years old. Their number in the human body is said to be hundreds of thousands and even reach millions. The three we mentioned above are the most vital. When they are unblocked through yoga and meditation the energy of *kundalini* rises from the base of the spine. *Nadis* are tasked with carrying the *prana*.

According to an old Vedic story, the five main powers of nature – speech, the mind, sight, and breath (*prana*), started to argue about which one was the most important. In order to resolve their argument, they made a decision. Each of them would leave the body and see whose absence would be missed the most. The first power that left was speech. However, the body kept flourishing even though it could not speak. The next power to leave was the eye. The body still kept flourishing even though it couldn't see. Then, the ear left, and the body continued to grow even though it was deaf. It was the mind's turn to leave and even unconscious, the body kept flourishing.

The only one left was the *prana*. However, when it started to leave, the body started to die. All the other powers were losing their life-force so fast that they could do nothing else but rush to the *prana*, admit its supremacy, and beg for it to stay. When the *prana* is absent, it is clear that it is the one that gives energy to all our faculties, and without it, they can't function.

To the physical body, they channel the air, nutrients, water, blood, and various other bodily fluids. They are similar to the bronchioles, veins, arteries, capillaries, lymph canals, etc. To the casual and subtle body, they channel the vital, mental, cosmic, intellectual, seminal, etc. energies which are collectively named *prana* and are vital for the spiritual aura, sensations, and consciousness.

Ida is connected with lunar energy. In Sanskrit, the word ida translates to "comfort". *Ida* has a feminine energy and a moonlike nature with a soothing effect. It spans from the left testicle to the left nostril. *Pingala* is connected with solar energy. In Sanskrit, it means "orange". It has masculine energy and a sun-like nature with a warm temperature, it spans from the right testicle to the right nostril. *Sashumna* is connected with both nostrils, free and open for the air to pass through. It connects the base chakra to the crown chakra and is essential in both Yoga and Tantra.

There are a number of techniques through which you can cleanse your *nadis* in order for the channel release of the life energy to all your seven chakras to take place. The most common and effective one is the alternate-nostril breathing. Below you will see how it happens:

- Sit comfortably in the yogic position *asana* as is shown in the picture.

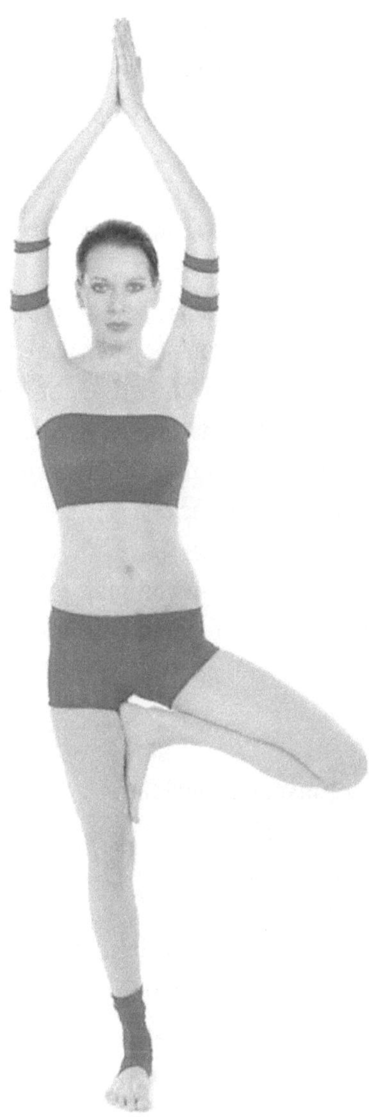

- If you are only a beginner in yoga, you may find it difficult to keep both your hands raised for the whole duration of the practice. To solve this issue you can place a bolster across your legs and use it in order to support your elbows.
- With one thumb, close your right nostril.

- Inhale through your left nostril.
- Then, close your left nostril with your ring finger.
- Open the right one and exhale slowly.
- Keep the right one open, inhale, close it, open, and exhale slowly through the left one.
- By now you have completed one cycle.
- Repeat this for 3 to 5 times and go back to normal breathing.

In Chinese tradition, the meridian system, also called channel network is found in traditional Chinese medicine and is the path through which the life-energy known as *"qi"* in this case flows. The meridians are not actually anatomical structures since there is no scientific proof of their existence. There are two categories corresponding to the meridian network:

- The *jingmai* or else meridian channels.
- The *luomai* or else the associated vessels.

The *jingmai* includes:

- The 12 tendinomuscular meridians
- The 12 divergent meridians
- The 12 principal meridians
- The 8 extraordinary vessels
- The *Huato* channel - a number of bilateral points located at the lower back discovered by the ancient physician Hua Tuo.

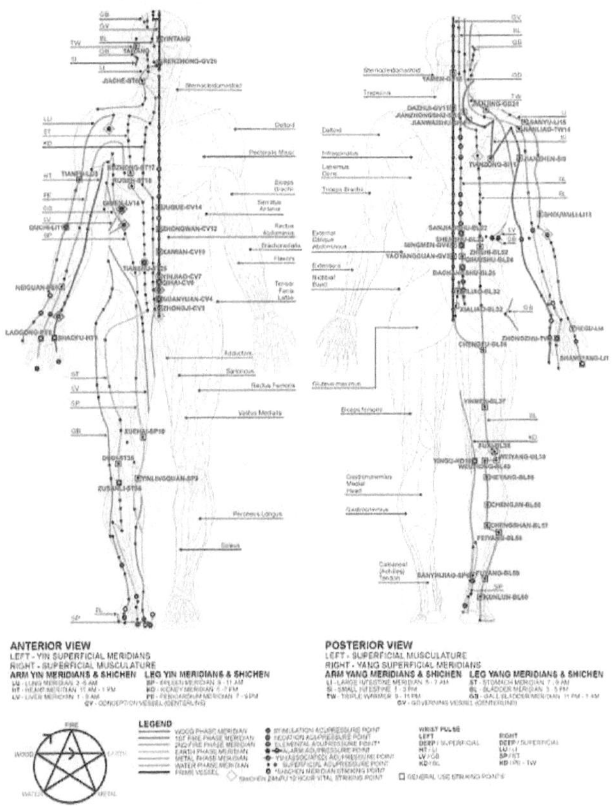

The associated vessels contain 15 essential arteries that connect the 12 principal meridians in several ways. They also contain a branching expanse of vessels similar to capillary that spread throughout the body, more specifically in the 12 cutaneous regions. The total count of the unique points on each meridian is 361, a number that matches the number of days in a year based on the moon calendar system. Keep in mind that this method does not take into consideration that the bulk of acupoints are bilateral which makes the total 670.

There are approximately 400 acupuncture points if we do not count the bilateral points twice which most of them are located along the major 20 pathways. However, in the Second Century AD, in China, 649 acupuncture points were recognized by counting the bilateral points twice. In this system, there are "12 Principal Meridians" with each one corresponding to a solid or a hollow organ and interacts with it. These 12 essential meridians are separated into Yin and Yang groups. The Yin meridians of the arm are:

- Pericardium.
- Lung.
- Heart.

The Yang meridians of the arm are:

- Small Intestine.
- Large Intestine.
- Triple Burner.

The Yin Meridians of the leg are:

- Liver.
- Kidney.
- Spleen.

The Yang meridians of the leg are:

- Gall Bladder.
- Stomach.
- Bladder.

There are also eight extraordinary meridians that are essential in the study of Chinese alchemy, *T'ai chi ch'uan*, and *Qigong*. These are different from the standard twelve meridians since they are believed to be storage or reservoirs vessels and not directly associated with the *Zang Fu* or else internal organs. The eight extraordinary vessels are:

- Conception Vessel - *Ren Mai*.
- Governing Vessel - *Du Mai*.
- Penetrating Vessel - *Chong Mai*.

- Girdle Vessel - *Dai Mai.*
- Yin linking vessel - *Yin Wei Mai.*
- Yang linking vessel - *Yang Wei Mai.*
- Yin Heel Vessel - *Yin Qiao Mai.*
- Yang Heel Vessel - *Yang Qiao Mai.*

The most common way for the meridians to be cleansed is through acupuncture which is essential to traditional Chinese medicine and it includes thin needles that are inserted into the body. Acupuncture has been characterized as pseudoscience due to the fact that the practices and theories of TCM do not come from scientific knowledge. There are many acupuncture variants that stem from different philosophies and its practices depend on the country that performs it. It is most commonly used for pain relief even though acupuncturists maintain that it can be used for a wider range of other conditions.

A typical session includes a person lying still while about five to 20 needles are inserted into his or her body. In most cases, the needles will remain in place for ten to 20 minutes. It can also be combined with the application of laser light, heat, or pressure. This form of alternative medicine is a non-invasive therapy that was developed in the early 20th century in Japan where they used an elaborate set of instruments that were not needles to treat children.

The most common tool for stimulation in acupuncture points is thin metal needles that penetrate the skin and are manually manipulated. There is also electro-acupuncture where the needle undergoes an electrical stimulation. The needles are most commonly made of stainless steel and are thus flexible and rusting or breaking is prevented. Usually, the needles are disposed after each session and when they are used again, they should be sterilized between applications.

Aside from acupuncture, there are several yoga poses that help with the cleansing and balance of the meridians. One example is the cat pose:

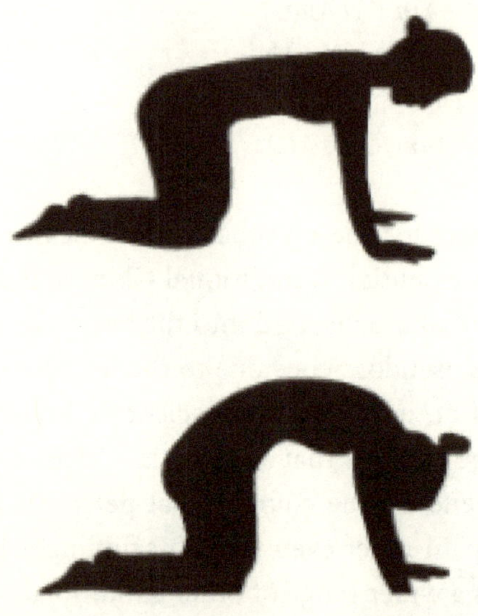

This pose is appropriate for the kidney meridian which helps to decompress the lower back. When in quadruped position, lower down your head and pull your navel towards your spine while arching your back as a cat does.

Another yoga pose is the cow pose. From the cat pose, you can then move into this one by having your head pointing towards the ceiling and leaving your back arched with your chest leaning forward. This pose helps with the stomach meridian that leads to improved digestion and cramping.

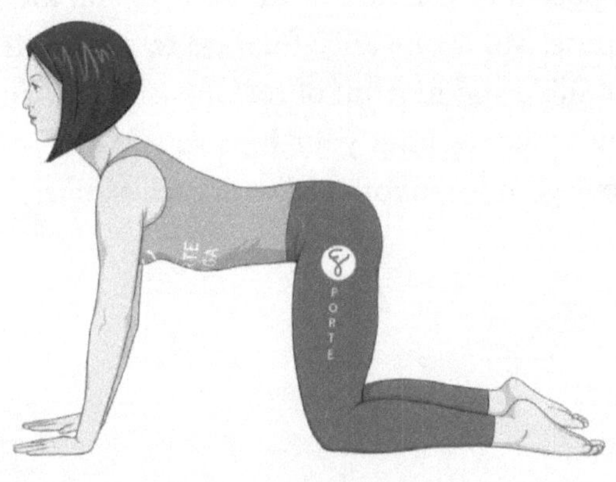

The seated wide leg pose helps with the kidney meridian. This is an appropriate pose if you are dealing with fear, shock, or if your adrenals are taxed and you feel exhausted. On a mat spread your legs wide to the level you are comfortable with on each side and move your torso forward as you breathe.

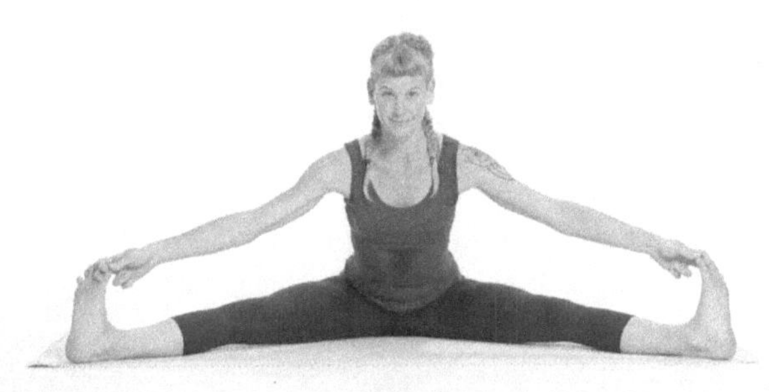

One last yoga pose that will help with the liver and kidney meridians is the pigeon pose. Move one knee forward to your wrist on the same side with your ankle and in front of the opposite hip. Then, slide your leg behind you while keeping your hips square and straight. Take a breath and move your torso forward with each exhale.

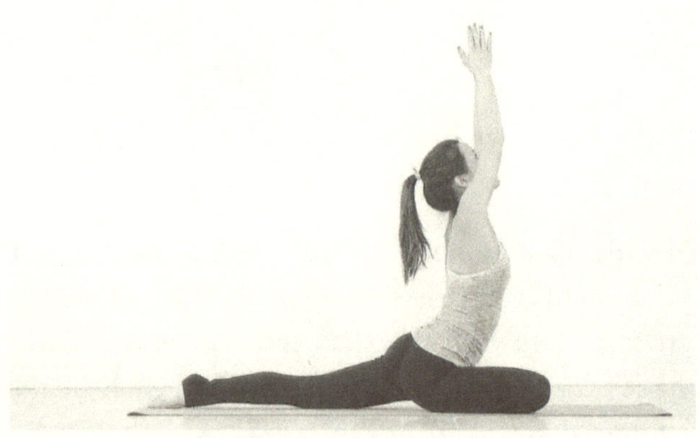

Our life force flows from specific lines of energy in this case the *nadis* or meridians to circulate all over the etheric body. By practicing the techniques, we mentioned above, you will be able to find the appropriate balance as well as the flow of the circulations in the channels of the body. They also help you with developing your resistance to the negative energies all around you.

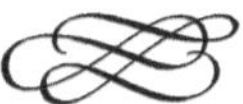

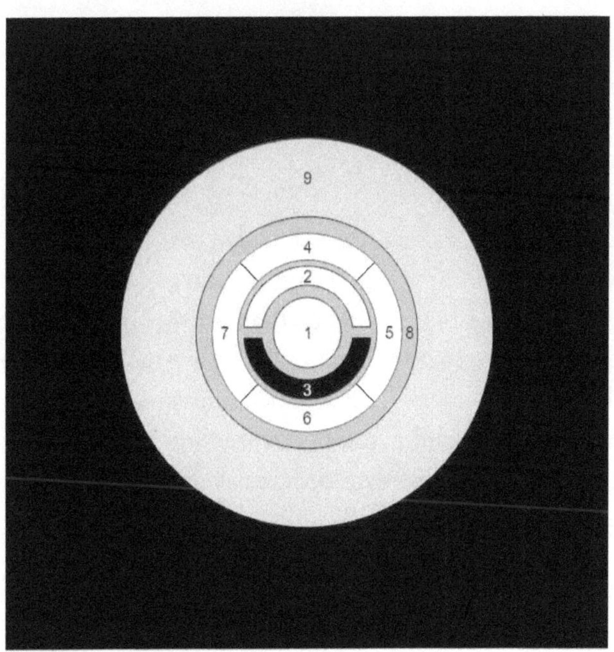

I n esoteric cosmology, there are different planes of existence which are conceived as a subtle region, state, or level of reality and each of these planes corresponds to some category, kind, or type of being. This concept can be traced in esoteric and religious teaching such as:

- *Shamanism.*
- *Ayyavazhi.*
- *Vedanta - Advaita Vedanta.*
- *Hermeticism.*
- *Neoplatonism.*
- *Gnosticism.*
- *Kashmir Shaivism.*
- *Sant Mat/Surat Shabd Yoga.*
- *Sufism.*
- *Druze.*
- *Kabbalah.*
- *Theosophy.*
- *Anthroposophy.*
- *Rosicrucianism* - Esoteric Christian.
- *Eckankar.*
- Ascended Master Teachings.

All of the above teachings promote the idea that there is a whole set of subtle worlds or planes which interpenetrate themselves from a center as well as the physical place that we live in, the solar system, and every physical structure of the universe. The interpenetration of all the planes comes to its climax in the universe seen as a dynamic, physically structured and evolutive expression coming from a series of steadily denser stages that progressively turn out to be more embodied and material.

According to esoteric teachings, this emanation originated from the dawn of the manifestation of the universe in The Supreme Being who sent from the unmanifested Absolute, something beyond our comprehension, the dynamic creative energy in the form of sound-vibration or else the World into the abyss which was space. The Supreme Being or The Great Architect of the Universe is a conception of God that has been debated by many Christian theologians and apologists. It is used as a designation within Freemasonry and stands for the neutral deity in whatever name and whichever form each member individually believes in.

Concepts of the planes of existence can be found in ancient traditions such as in India with the *bhuvanas* and *lokas*. According to Hindu cosmology, there are many worlds or *lokas* that are similar to both the states of meditation and traditional cosmology. In esoteric conceptions, the alchemists of the Middle ages tried to cloak their proposed ideas about the birth of the universe through a hermetic language filled with esoteric phrases, signs, and words so as to not be understood by those who were not initiated into the ways of alchemy.

The Rosicrucian alchemist Jan Baptist van Helmont, wrote in his *"Physica"* in 1633, *"Ad huc spiritum incognitum Gas voco"* which translates to "This hitherto unknown Spirit I call Gas." Also, in the same work, he says, "This vapor which I have called Gas is not far removed from the Chaos the ancients spoke of". The metaphysical terms planes were made popular in the late 19th century by the Theosophy of H. P. Blavatsky, who in *The Secret Doctrine* proposed a complex cosmology composed of seven planes and sub-planes which was based on the synthesis of Western and Eastern ideas. From there, the term was used in later esoteric systems like that of Alice Bailey who greatly influenced the shaping of the New Age movement.

The belief of most cosmologists today is that the universe expanded from a singularity about 13.8 billion years ago in an event called the Big Bang which means that space was created the moment of the big bang and ever since it has expanded and created the galaxies within it. On the other hand, the expansion in esoteric cosmology refers to the emanation of steadily denser spheres or planes from the spiritual reality which was referred to by the Greeks as *The One*, until the most material and lowest world is reached. According to the *Rosicrucians*, there is another difference which is that there is no void or empty space. More specifically:

"The space is Spirit in its attenuated form; while the matter is crystallized space or Spirit. Spirit in manifestation is dual, that which we see as Form is the negative manifestation of Spirit - crystallized and inert. The positive pole of Spirit manifests as Life, galvanizing the negative Form into action, but both Life and Form originated in Spirit, Space, Chaos! On the other hand, Chaos is not a state which has existed in the past and has now entirely disappeared. It is all around us at the present moment. Were it not that old forms - having outlived their usefulness - are constantly being resolved back into that Chaos, which is also as constantly giving birth to new forms, there could be no progress; the work of evolution would cease and stagnation would prevent the possibility of advancement." - Heindel, Max, The Rosicrucian Cosmo-Conception (Chapter XI: The Genesis and Evolution of our Solar System), 1909.

So, according to esoteric authors, psychics, and occult teachings, there are seven planes of existence. The first one is the physical plane or physical universe, and physical World in emanationist metaphysics from Hermeticism, Theosophy, Neoplatonism, and Hinduism refers to the visible reality of time, matter, energy, and space. This is the densest or lowest of all planes of existence, according to esoteric cosmology and Occultism. Based on the Theosophists, the etheric plane follows the physical plane and both of them are connected to create the first plane. Also, Theosophy maintains that when our physical body dies, the etheric body survives and the soul form into an astral body residing on the astral plane.

The astral plane or else the astral world or space is the place where our consciousness goes after we physically perish. Based on occult philosophy, each and every one of us has an astral body. This plane is supported by neo-platonic, esoteric, oriental, and medieval philosophies as well as mystery religions. It is the plane of the planetary spheres that the soul crosses in its astral body as it goes to be born and after it dies. It is generally said to be populated by spirits, immaterial being, and angels. Throughout the Renaissance, Paraceisians, alchemists, philosophers, and *Rosicrusians* continued to debate the nature of the astral plane in connection with the divine and the Earth.

Based on occult teachings, someone can visit the astral plane through astral projection, mantra, meditation, lucid dreaming, and near-death experience. There are many people training to use the astral vehicle that separates their consciousness from the physical body at will. According to occultist George Arundale:

"In the astral world exists temporarily all those physical entities, men and animals, for whom sleep involves a separation of the physical body for a time from the higher bodies. While we "sleep", we live in our astral bodies, either fully conscious and active, or partly conscious and semi-dormant, as the case may be, according to our evolutionary growth; when we "wake", the physical and the higher bodies are inter-locked again, and we cease to be inhabitants of the astral world."

Paramhansa Yogananda, in the book "Autobiography of a Yogi" presents us with details about the astral plane that were learned by his resurrected guru *Swami Sri* Yukteswar Giri. These details include that almost all people after their death enter the astral plane. In this plane, they work on the seeds of past karma through astral incarnations and if it is needed, they return to earthly incarnations to refine further. The moment a person has achieved the meditative state of *nirvikalpa samadhi* in an astral incarnation or an earthly one, the soul will move forward to the "illumined astral planet" of *Hiranyaloka*. After this stage, the soul will move upward to more casual and subtle spheres and the following incarnations will allow them to refine further the final unification.

Based on the Hermeticism, Rosicrucian, New Age, Theosophical, and Aurobindonian thought, the mental plane or else the world of thought is the third-lowest plane, the universal or macrocosmic plane or reality that is constructed purely of thought as opposed to the post-modern and Western secular modernist thought. In esoteric and occult cosmology consciousness and thoughts are not simply a result of brain functioning but have their own universal and objective reality which is independent of the physical.

This is the reality that is only a part of a sequence of different planes of existence. In such similar explanations of reality and cosmology, the mental plane is found between the astral plane which is located below, and the higher spiritual realms of existence above. The mental plane is separated into seven sub-planes. According to Charles Webster Leadbeater, a member of the Theosophical Society, an author on occult subjects and co-founder with J. I. Wedgwood of the Liberal Catholic Church:

"In the mental world one formulates a thought and it is instantly transmitted to the mind of another without any expression in the form of words. Therefore on that plane language does not matter in the least; but helpers working in the astral world, who have not yet the power to use the mental vehicle."

In Hindu occultism the mental plane is made up of two divisions, the first is the lower division that is known to us as heaven and the upper-division known to us as the casual plane. According to Sivaya Subramuniyaswami also known as Gurudeva by his followers, was the 162nd head of the Nandinatha Sampradaya's Kailasa Parampara and Guru at Kauai's Hindu Monastery which is a 382-acre (155 ha) temple-monastery complex on Hawaii's Garden Island,

"The causal plane is the world of light and blessedness, the highest of heavenly regions, extolled in the scriptures of all faiths. It is the foundation of existence, the source of visions, the point of conception, the apex of creation. The causal plane is the abode of Lord Siva and his entourage of *Mahadevas* and other highly evolved souls who exist in their own self-effulgent form—radiant bodies of centillions of quantum light particles."

Moving on to the *Buddhic* plane, it is the realm of pure consciousness. Based on Theosophy, this plane has the privilege to develop *Buddhic* consciousness which translates to people solving any issues with the ego and becoming unselfish. According to Charles Webster Leadbeater, in the *Buddhic* plane, we cast off the illusion of self and enter a state of unity. Annie Besant, a British socialist, theosophist, women's rights activist, writer, orator, educationist, and philanthropist, defined this plane as:

"Persistent, conscious, spiritual awareness. This is the full consciousness of the *Buddhic* or intuitional level. This is the perceptive consciousness which is the outstanding characteristic of the Hierarchy. The life focus of the man shifts to the *Buddhic* plane. This is the fourth or middle state of consciousness."

The spiritual plane is divided into various sub-planes and on these reside more advanced in status and development than humans, spiritual beings. Based on metaphysical thought the aim of the spiritual plane is to achieve spiritual experience and knowledge.

The Divine plane is the home of all souls, where they are born, and then travel down to the lower planes. However, the souls will return to the divine plane where they can open to the conscious communication with the divine sphere known as the Absolute and gain knowledge about the true form of reality. This is the plane where *Om* and *Brahman*, or in other words the creative world, exists.

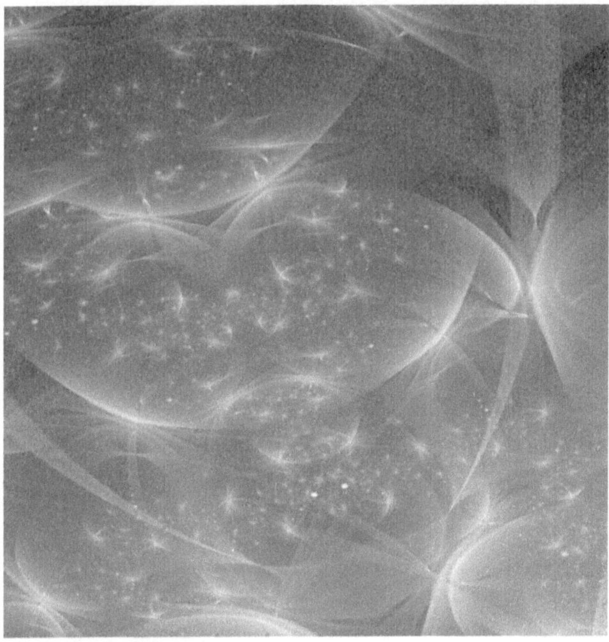

The logic plane is the highest plane and is total oneness, where we become united with God. There is also the *Monadic* plane where the Holy Spirit or *monad* is said to exist. In Buddhism, the world is constructed by 31 planes of existence that a person can be reborn into and are separated into 3 realms. These realms and worlds are:

The Immaterial World - *arupa-loka.*

- Neither-perception-nor-non-perception - *nevasaññanasaññayatanupaga deva.*
- Nothingness - *akiñcaññayatanupaga deva.*
- Infinite Consciousness - *viññanañcayatanupaga deva.*
- Infinite Space - *akasanañcayatanupaga deva.*

The Fine-Material World - *rupa-loka.*

- Peerless devas- *akanittha deva.*
- Clear-sighted devas - *sudassi deva.*
- Beautiful devas - *sudassa deva.*
- Untroubled devas - *atappa deva.*
- Devas not Falling Away - *aviha deva.*
- Unconscious beings – *asaññasatta.*
- Very Fruitful devas - *vehapphala deva.*
- Devas of Refulgent Glory - *subhakinna deva.*
- Devas of Unbounded Glory - *appamanasubha deva.*
- Devas of Limited Glory - *parittasubha deva.*
- Devas of Streaming Radiance - *abhassara deva.*
- Devas of Unbounded Radiance - *appamanabha deva.*
- Devas of Limited Radiance - *parittabha deva.*
- Great Brahmas - *Maha brahma.*
- Ministers of Brahma - *brahma-purohita deva.*
- Retinue of Brahma - *brahma-parisajja deva.*

The Sensuous World - *kama-loka.*

- Devas Wielding Power over the Creation of Others -
  paranimmita-vasavatti deva.
- Devas Delighting in Creation - *nimmanarati deva.*
- Yama devas - *yama deva.*
- The Thirty-three Gods - *tavatimsa deva.*
- Devas of the Four Great Kings - *catumaharajika deva.*
- Human beings - *manussa loka.*

States of Deprivation - *Apaya*

- *Asuras – asura.*
- Hungry Shades/Ghosts - *peta loka.*
- Animals - *tiracchana yoni.*
- Hell – *niraya.*

The astral world is the place we come from birth and will return when we perish. Connecting with the astral world is very important because this is where you will realize the freedom of your true nature. You came from the astral world to begin with, in the form of a cloaked soul and due to the fact that you do not reside there now all memories you had, have been lost and the misery you go through in this world persists.

When you connect with the astral space you will be able to learn how to heal as well as all the causes of diseases and suffering. There people discover the secret to their existence and most importantly what happens after death, a question that cannot be answered even by science. You will learn how to live in the material world without having to lose your divine connection. There are no limitations in the astral world as opposed to our material world.

When the soul leaves the astral world in order to be born on earth, the human baby finds himself or herself confined and restricted in the womb of the mother and wishes to get out, but this is not possible and the baby has to wait for nine months. Then, the baby is subjected to being helpless during infancy and as the baby grows and becomes an adolescence, he or she is forced to fight and find a path through emotions and passions which make him or her feel out of control and as a result, goes through all kinds of misery. Then this person marries and struggles to support the growing family but perhaps this person may be happy for a while, however, as this person gets older the machine that holds him together, his body, begins to fail and then he or she perishes. This is the what in Hinduism is material limitations.

If you were able to connect with the astral world, you would be able to know that material existence is only a shadow of the astral world, it is only a result of it. The blueprints of everything that exists in the physical universe have been premade in the astral world as is the case with all the forces and forms in nature including the human body. However, the astral world is not the final liberating experience the soul will be able to achieve. This will be achieved only if it realizes it is one with the creator himself, but the soul will keep going in an effort to disengage from the material world and into the higher awareness of the finer astral existence.

Now, you may be wondering how one can connect with that higher plane. You should keep in mind that in your thoughts you have always been there, however, just because you have been so identified with the physical perceptions of your thoughts, the astral world and its powers have changed you. Your soul visits the astral world while you fall asleep, but you are not aware of it. So connecting with the astral plane may take time but not because you have to be taught all over again how to connect with it, but because it may take time to practice, first with awakening your Third Eye, which is one of the ways to connect with the astral plane as well as start practicing all the other methods that can lead you to a safe and secure connection with the astral plane.

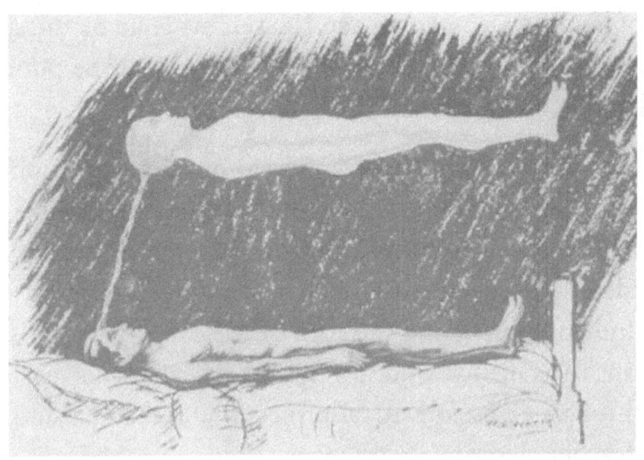

One of the best-known ways to connect to the astral plane is through astral projection or astral travel. Astral projection happens when the mind leaves the body and is set free to explore the parallel astral plane. From there you can visit any place in the universe and meet with various other consciousnesses that also travel to the astral plane including someone you may already know. Astral travel is used in *esoterism* to describe an out of body experience that is done intentionally and validates the existence of a consciousness or soul named the "astral body" and it is separate from the physical body as well as able to travel outside and throughout the universe.

Astral projection is not a new idea and dates back to ancient times and is found in many cultures. However, the term astral projection was promoted by Theosophists in the 19th century. Many people have reported going through experiences similar to astral projection and were able to initiate them through various hypnotic and hallucinogenic means such as self-hypnosis, but there is no scientific evidence to support the existence of a consciousness or else a soul that is different from the neural activity or that someone can consciously leave their body and observe as a result, astral projection has been widely characterized as pseudoscience.

Based on medieval, classical, and renaissance Neoplatonism, Theosophist, Hermeticism, and Rosicrucian thought, the astral body links the rational soul to the physical body with the astral plane being a world of light between Earth and Heaven made up by the spheres of the stars and the planets. These spheres are said to be populated by spirits, demons, and angels.

The concept of soul travel is found in various other religions such as ancient Egyptian teachings where the soul has the ability to move outside of the physical body using the *ka* or else the subtle body. Similar ideas are presented in the ancient Hindu scriptures with modern Indians supporting the idea of the astral projection such as Paramahansa Yogananda who saw Swami Pranabananda performing a miracle through a possible astral projection. Meher Baba, the Indian spiritual teacher, described astral projection:

"In the advancing stages leading to the beginning of the path, the aspirant becomes spiritually prepared for being entrusted with free use of the forces of the inner world of the astral bodies. He may then undertake astral journeys in his astral body, leaving the physical body in sleep or wakefulness. The astral journeys that are taken unconsciously are much less important than those undertaken with full consciousness and as a result of deliberate volition. This implies conscious use of the astral body. Conscious separation of the astral body from the outer vehicle of the gross body has its own value in making the soul feel its distinction from the gross body and in arriving at fuller control of the gross body. One can, at will, put on and take off the external gross body as if it were a cloak, and use the astral body for experiencing the inner world of the astral and for undertaking journeys through it, if and when necessary. The ability to undertake astral journeys, therefore, involves a considerable expansion of one's scope for experience. It brings opportunities for promoting one's own spiritual advancement, which begins with the involution of consciousness."

The ability of the soul to leave the body intentionally while a person is sleeping and travel to the different planes of heaven is also known as soul travel. This is taught in Surat Shabd Yoga where it is achieved by mantra repetition and meditation techniques. Practicing the various techniques to develop your astral projection and your out of body exploration can be very satisfying and enjoyable. Throughout history, nearly every Mystic order and religious group has created a method or system to explore the world beyond the material limits. We will present to you out of body techniques that separated into five categories:

- Dream conversion.
- Hypnosis.
- Sound.
- Visualization.
- Affirmations.

You should always remember that if you wish to practice astral projection and connect to the astral plane, one of the most important decisions you will have to make is to select the appropriate technique for you. For instance, if you are able to visualize well, you should concentrate on the visualization technique. Generally, you need to select the technique which makes you more comfortable and keep practicing on it. If you are finding it difficult to visualize, then you can concentrate on the affirmations technique. Most importantly do not underestimate your abilities, especially when you keep an open mind to new perceptions and experiences since this is when they will certainly occur.

Below are listed some basic out of body exploration principles to remember while practicing the techniques we're about to show you:

- We are all spiritual beings, so we use only our temporary biological bodies to express ourselves and gain experience.
- So, since the body is only a tool, it is only natural to be able to separate our soul from it and experience our nonphysical self.
- When we go through out of body experiences, we normally transfer or shift our awareness from our physical body to the higher frequencies of energy vehicles.
- We are responsible for creating our individual reality through

the way we manage and focus our personal energy, something that applies to all energy levels of the universe.
- All that we experience has been manifested, influenced, and arranged by our subconscious and conscious thoughts.

Dreams are believed to be the doorway to astral projection or out of body exploration. Many people have reported the dreams to them are the natural way to shift their awareness from their physical state of consciousness to experiencing as well as recognizing other states of consciousness. From the ancient to today's world different cultures and societies all over the world have recognized that dreams are an essential doorway that leads to a different world. For instance, the importance of dreams is depicted in the oldest recorded writings such as The Egyptian Book of the Dead, The Bible, The Upanishads, and The Koran.

If we use them properly, dreams can trigger out of body exploration. One of the most effective ways to signal or initiate astral projection is to be lucid or aware within the dream. This can be done by altering the attitude we have towards our dreams. For example, we need to acknowledge how important dreams are in our daily life. You should treat your dreams as insights as well as messages that come from your subconscious mind. Think of them as a true form of communication which is as real as physical experiences.

You can start a daily dream journal in which you can record every detail of your dream that you can remember, however small. Writing in your journal should be done immediately when you wake up or you can even use a tape recorder. You should also record your emotions, sensations, and feelings you experienced during your dreams. Expressing firmly your need for increased awareness and clarity within your dreams will help in the process of experiencing an astral projection. When you find yourself in a near-sleep state, firmly decide that your whole conscious awareness should be present in your dreams. You can make a verbal commitment to yourself which you will recognize, consciously experience, and recall in every single one of your dreams.

Then, repeat this firm decision to yourself before you go to sleep each night. For instance, you can repeat "as I drift off to sleep, I am aware" or "I am aware in my dreams". As you repeat your affirmations make sure they are positive and firm and fully expect your decision to be implemented. As is the case with astral projection, focus your intellectual and emotional energy into each affirmation because it is essential to focus on them and let them be your last conscious thought as you fall asleep. This transfer of awareness can be done relatively quickly so always remember that it is important to keep calm and enjoy any changes in your environment, location, energy, or perspective.

Be willing to accept and recognize the entire process that takes place in your dream. How we respond when our awareness is fully present in our dreams is of utmost importance. Keep in mind that lucid or vivid dreams do not necessarily translate in out of body experiences but rather are a psychological manifestation that is closely related to an internal projection. The bizarre events that happen in our dreams are actually creations of our subconscious mind and have been particularly designed to get our attention. Once you fully commit to exploring out of body experiences the first step towards achieving this commitment is going through lucid dreaming and as a result, they become a regular event.

If you experience lucid dreams, you should be certain that you are on the right path to achieve astral projection because our subconscious mind is doing everything it can to help us achieve this goal of an intentional astral projection. This is why writing down your goals is important because the more focus you place on your goal the more your subconscious mind will offer you its help. Lucid dreams can be anything that seems out of the ordinary such as unusual people or surroundings, strange shapes, colors, animals, pets, or buildings, anything that seems inappropriate or illogical, generally things that are obviously not normal. The key to succeed in your goal of intentional astral projection and to connect to the astral plane is your conscious acknowledgment and response to your lucid dreams. Even if you see a regular animal or pet turn into an eagle, lion, or a dragon you need to dedicate your complete attention to the dream no matter how strange it may seem.

Once your attention is focused on the anomaly of the dream say out loud anything that will show your conscious acknowledgment such as "I am awake in my dream" or "I am fully present in my dream". Then, be prepared for the movement or transition of your consciousness from your dream state to your subtle body. It is also very common to wake up in a vibrational state while you are still inside your physical body or you are feeling out of sync with your physical body. The solution to such occurrences is to remain calm and direct your awareness away from your physical body. This whole process is very natural since dreams are designed and created to help us in our personal development. It is your choice to recognize them and use them appropriately or simply ignore them. No matter what you decide, your subconscious mind will keep sending you dreams with hidden messages to help you.

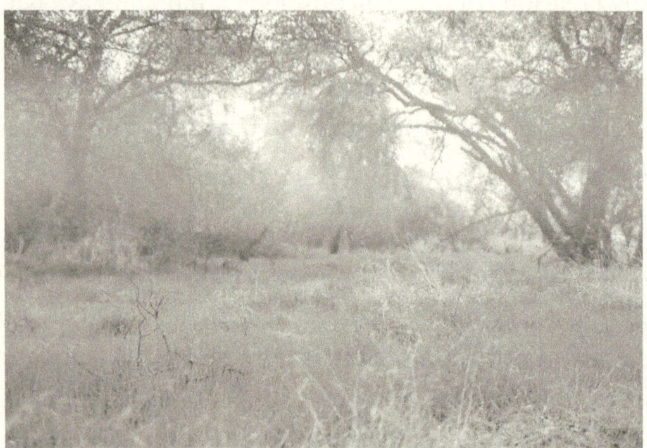

Below is a list of steps guiding you on how to respond to dream awareness:

- Be aware of any illogical or strange events, objects, or
  situations within your dream.

- Focus your attention as much as possible on these strange occurrences within your dream.
- Express verbally the strange object or event within your dream such as: "I don't have a castle," or "I can't fly".
- As you become increasingly lucid or else conscious within your dream express verbally that you know that you are dreaming.
- Prepare yourself for a quick shift in your awareness. It is plausible for you to awaken within a vibrational state that includes unusual sounds combined with vibrations felt in your entire body.
- Do not lose your calm and let these inner sensations continue as you direct immediately your complete attention away from your physical body.
- Maintain all your thoughts on the idea of transferring yourself to a different area in your home.
- It is extremely important to keep your complete awareness away from your physical body because any thoughts that have to do with your physical body will lead you back to it.
- Return your awareness to your body in a firm manner and be specific about your demands for immediate action.

Below you will also find the number of signals your dream is sending you:

- Seeing or feeling yourself near a vehicle of any type.
- Seeing or feeling yourself in a vehicle of any type such as a boat, automobile, or plane. You may also experience in your dream the motion of a vehicle or a boating adventure.
- Recognizing a difference in your everyday environment such as your home becoming a castle, a log cabin, or a palace.
- Recognizing any change in the construction, location, or color of your surroundings.
- Having feelings and sensations as well as experiences that resemble paralysis, abnormal sounds, energy surges, or numbness.

- Recognizing unusual situations, abilities, or events such as the ability to float, move in abnormal ways, or the ability to fly.
- Having the experience of sinking or falling which includes moving up and down the stairs, escalators, or elevators.
- Being in an environment that rapidly changes such as things that disappear or appear quickly.
- Recognizing conflict or a problem, for example, driving fast on a long road and the brakes are not working.
- Being presented with an opening of any kind such as a tunnel or a bridge which in your dream translates in helping you to overcome a barrier or an obstacle, for instance, a river or a wall.
- Being in the presence of a companion that acts as your guide and often this guide remains out of your vision even though they are next to you.
- Seeing multiple levels of any kind such as office buildings, parking garages, or ships.
- Reading a computer program or a book that has to do with advanced or unusual information.

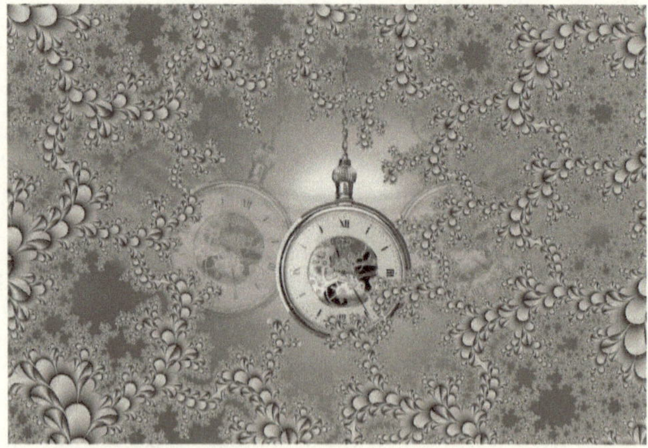

Today hypnosis has risen in popularity as a tool for self-improvement. It is most commonly used as a therapy for modifying behavior that has to do with sports improvement, weight control, memory enhancement, stress release, as well as treating phobias and fears. The latest developments in hypnosis have shown it to be used for past life regression with growing numbers of published hypnotic regressions getting information from past centuries such as events, names, places, and dates. Modern hypnosis is used to allow people to visit a previous physical life and during such sessions, the individual may experience, uncover, and resolve a present phobia, fear, or problem by finding its source.

It is believed that these past life regressions present a tendency to undergo an out-of-body state of awareness and it most commonly happens at the transition stage between physical lives. As a result, hypnosis could be a useful tool for inducing voluntarily out of body experiences. In the past decade, hypnosis has offered many benefits, especially in the area of astral projection such as:

- Hypnosis can effectively create the appropriate mental state for the exploration of astral projection by keeping your mind alert and your body relaxed.
- It can assist in the elimination, reduction, and control of conscious and subconscious fears, limits, and blocks that relate to astral projection.
- Hypnosis can assist in the dream conversion process by triggering a fully conscious astral projection. For instance, by saying "Sleep initiates my astral projection experience," you can enhance and reinforce your ability to respond positively in your out of body experiences.
- Hypnosis can be used for the enhancement of meditative skills, as well as concentration, and visualization.

Self-hypnosis is a powerful tool for your self-improvement since limits and fears are often programmed subconsciously within us. While internally we may have accepted a specific concept of abilities and ourselves, subconsciously we have placed limits on our potential and abilities. Such limits are what blocks us from our true potential, it is as if they have placed a wall around true selves. One effective way to break these self-accepted fears and limits is to directly confront them at the source which can be done through hypnosis. It offers us access to our subconscious mind and to find the solution to our limits and fears. We can also program our subconscious mind to succeed in anything including astral travel.

You can use a self-hypnosis script at home but make sure you never use it when driving a car or in other inappropriate situations. You can work with a professional. If you choose to work with a self-hypnosis script, while you record it, make sure you have the time in order to speak slowly and with a relaxed voice. During breaks between phrases, pause for about two seconds, and try to be consistent. Try to not speed up as you record and be relaxed. When using the script make sure you are comfortable and, in an area, where you will feel safe to go through astral travel. Make sure there will be no disturbances.

Using sound to initiate astral projection has been practiced throughout ancient times dating back thousands of years. For instance, Tibetan shamans and monks are well known for using chimes, bells, and chants to induce their meditative states. In recent years, the use of mantras and chanting has become an integral part of the meditation process. Repeating certain sounds is widely accepted and known as a method to improve and enhance a person's attention span.

Let us see a classic sound technique practiced by Tibetan monks:

- Relax completely and take several deep breaths.
- Make yourself comfortable in your astral travel area.
- Close your eyes and focus on the area of your head just above the crown.
- Concentrate your whole awareness above your head until you feel all your body's sensations disappear.
- As you feel all your physical sensations disappearing, softly intone the sound *Om* seven times.

- Let the sound travel through the top of your head.
- Utter the sound *Om* in your mind seven times.
- Be aware of the nature of the sound in your mind.
- Let the sound rise to the top of your head.
- Keep your attention on the core of the resonance and let the sound rise slowly towards the ceiling.
- Feel your awareness rise with the sound and become one with it as your body relaxes more.
- Feel your awareness rise along with the sound.
- Merge with the *Om* resonance.
- Flow with the sound and enjoy it.
- Leave your physical body asleep and rest as your attention is solely focused on the rising sound.
- As your body falls asleep do not shift your focus from the rising sound.

You can use this technique with an astral projection induction sound tape. If you follow an external sound system, do not forget to focus your whole attention upon the internal sounds due to the fact that external sounds are only designed as a reinforcement of your own voice.

Another popular technique on approaching astral projection and connecting with the astral plane is keeping your focus solely outside your body and upon an object, place, or a person located away from you. This is otherwise known as the visualization technique. It doesn't matter if you select a physical object or a person, make sure they are easy to visualize and are of interest to you. For many people the visualization of a person they love and are away from is very effective. You should visualize this person that you wish was with you in as much detail as possible. It is recommended that you are emotionally involved with that person and not have an imaginary relationship. Let that person absorb you to their presence and feel along with that person.

Keep the visualization of that person for as long as you can and allow your physical body to relax and fall asleep. It is essential for you to keep a detailed image of that person as you go to sleep. Then, as you drift off, try to enhance your visual and emotional connection to that person for as long as you can. This method works best as a bedtime visualization. The more emotionally attached you are, the more effective the process will be.

Also, the ability to maintain and focus your awareness away from your physical body is boosted if you bring your attention to a certain place or an object. It would be preferable to find objects and places found in your home. Select three physical targets that you can easily visualize. Each of the targets should be in the same area of your home and in a different room than you commonly use for your astral travel. After you choose your targets, move to each one, and examine their every detail by studying them from different perspectives. Do not rush the examination because you need to memorize the feelings and sights connected with each of your target areas. Be aware of your senses as you walk, especially of your touch and sight. Repeat the walk to these targets several times so as to remember every little detail of the area.

Focus on everything such as textures, weight, density, and colors. Enjoy all the sensory input that you can. It is essential for this technique to maintain your focus away from your physical body as it goes to sleep. To make sure that you will get the most out of this exercise, repeat your visual and physical walk through every day for one month. Be interested in each target since this method can also increase your visualization and concentration skills. Many people choose personal items that also have sentimental value. Once you have selected your targets, stick with them, repeating your visualization can enhance its effectiveness dramatically.

Affirmations can also induce astral projection since they have proven how effective they are for the past four decades. They are an integral part of self-improvement methods all over the world. As an affirmation, we define a positive and strong comment about yourself in the present. It is a method that solidifies an idea or thought about us and when they are used in the right way, they are very effective. An affirmation can be for instance, "I deserve love" or "I am a happy person". They should always be uttered in a positive statement.

It is a fact that our minds are constantly flooded with thoughts and our thoughts influence our non-physical and physical reality. Our emotional, physical, and intellectual state of consciousness is a direct result of the way we think. With affirmations, we will be able to counteract some of our negative thoughts that we have accepted as reality. Replacing negativity with positive and fresh thoughts is the result of practicing with affirmations and reprogramming ourselves to achieve personal success.

You can repeat affirmations aloud, silently, in writing, or in the form of a rhyme or a song. When practicing for astral projection, people usually repeat them silently with an emphasis on the time before sleep. The aim is to have your whole attention turned to your desire for an instant out of the body experience as you fall asleep. To perform this method right your need to do four things:

- Increase progressively and as much as you can the intellectual and emotional intensity of your affirmations before you go to sleep.
- Repeat your affirmations up until the moment you fall asleep without stopping.
- Make sure your final thoughts before you fall asleep are your astral travel affirmations.
- Think of the affirmations as your personal commitment that you truly wish to experience.
- Be as open as possible to get the immediate results of your chosen affirmations.

Below are a few examples of affirmations about astral travel:

- Now I am astral traveling!
- I enjoy astral projection now!
- I consciously experience an astral travel journey. Now!
- I am aware even as my body is sleeping!

- I consciously leave my physical body after it falls asleep.
- I am more than my physical body.
- I remain aware of my astral projection as my body sleeps.
- I float above my body.
- Now I am separating from my body.
- Now I go through an astral travel experience.

Affirmations can be very useful for astral projection in the following ways:

- You affirm the clarity of your perception when you are having an out of body experience.
- You declare your instant intentions to go through an astral travel journey.
- You reduce fear and control.
- You enhance the process of dream conversion and memory recall.
- You reinforce and enhance all of the astral projection techniques.
- You control your thoughts before and throughout astral travel experiences.
- You help in the removal of limiting and negative beliefs and concepts that have to do with astral travel.
- You go through an effective method to reprogram your subconscious and succeed.
- You improve your ability to separate from your physical body during astral travel.

Connecting with the astral plane can be a transformative experience for you. Astral projection being the most common path to the astral plane, keep in mind that the results of astral travel can vary from one person to another. Transferring your awareness rapidly from your physical to your nonphysical body can be a startling experience if you are not prepared for it. For this reason, you should maintain a positive response to any abrupt change of perception, location, or viewpoint, an essential requirement if you wish to undergo a successful and controlled astral travel experience.

Below your will find a list with the most commonly reported experiences after an astral travel technique:

- Standing, lying, or floating outside your physical body.
- Seeing the energy version of yourself sitting or lying within your physical body. This may come along with intense vibrations throughout your whole energy body.
- You may feel out of sync with your physical body.
- Sitting or standing on one of the target areas you chose and observing the new environment.
- A rapid shift of awareness. In this case, you should enjoy the new perception and remain calm.
- Experiencing a lucid dream where you are extremely aware of your environment.
- Experiencing non-physical environments that are completely different from your daily one. Make sure to remain calm as well as enjoy and explore your new surroundings.

Practicing one of the above methods, the one that fits you best, will help you in initiating an astral projection experience that will connect you to the beautiful world that is the astral plane where you will be at peace and have access to unlimited wisdom. For many people, the ultimate and most sacred goal is to be reunited with their spiritual essence or else the higher self.

This experience has been praised over the centuries for its ability to impact liberation and enlightenment. Many teachers and writers have tried to describe this experience but how could someone describe precisely what happens beyond our known world? For this reason, connecting to the astral plane will be a unique experience for you. What better way to help you further understand the importance of developing your connection with the astral plane than in the words of Paramahansa Yogananda:

"From the astral world we come at birth, and there we shall return at death. Someone asked me why we should try to connect with the astral world now. To this, I reply, "Because that is where you will realize the freedom of your true nature. You were there as a soul cloaked in an astral form to start with; and because you are not there now and have lost that memory is why all your misery persists. By entering that other world, we learn the causes and healing of all suffering and diseases. We discover the secret of our existence — what happens after death, and where we were before birth, and how to live in the material world without losing our divine connection"

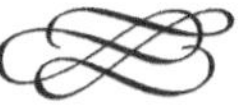

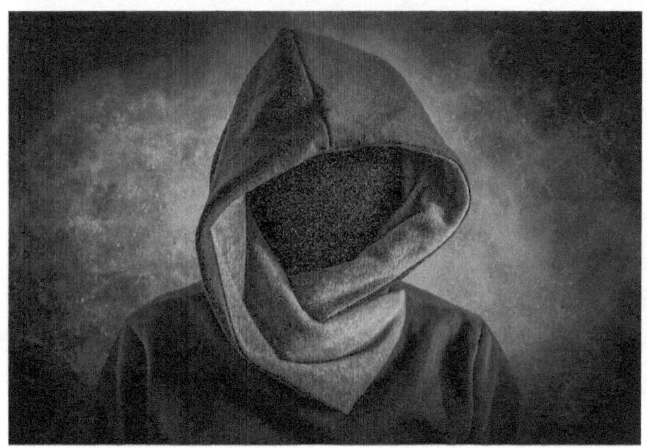

Psychics have existed and been consulted for thousands of years. For example, ancient Egyptians turned to the seers in order to communicate with their deities, Native Americans along with various indigenous people honor, and keep doing so, shamans, the people who have a connection with animal and earth spirits. Leaders in ancient Greece consulted the oracles of Delphi who were gifted to receive messages from the god Apollo. In ancient China, various divinatory practices were developed such as face reading, palmistry, and I Ching.

Communicating with spirits was stigmatized and banned in the 13th century, during the spread of Christianity. Then, religious leaders believed that psychics were communicating with the devil. As a result, indigenous practices and beliefs were forbidden by colonists during the 16th century when various cultures were made to follow the institutionalized religion. However, particular figures such as Nostradamus, who made certain serious predictions, rose in popularity worldwide.

Spiritualism gained ground in the mid-19th century. During this time, its followers organized public meetings to demonstrate psychics connecting with the spirit world and delivered messages to the people present. Those messages were proof of the presence of their loved ones in the afterlife. Nowadays, psychics are not restrained and are allowed to openly work. It comes as no surprise if a person's friends, colleague, or a family member consults regularly with psychics. Some very well-known psychics are Theresa Caputo, John Henry, James Van Praagh, and Sylvia Brown.

Despite the fact that psychics have been dismissed by the scientific community, their popularity has only grown. Besides, how could you explain something that can't be explained? How do you measure something that has existed for thousands of years? How can you prove the existence of a soul? At some point, with the rising focus on quantum mechanics, it is possible that the psychic phenomena will be proven.

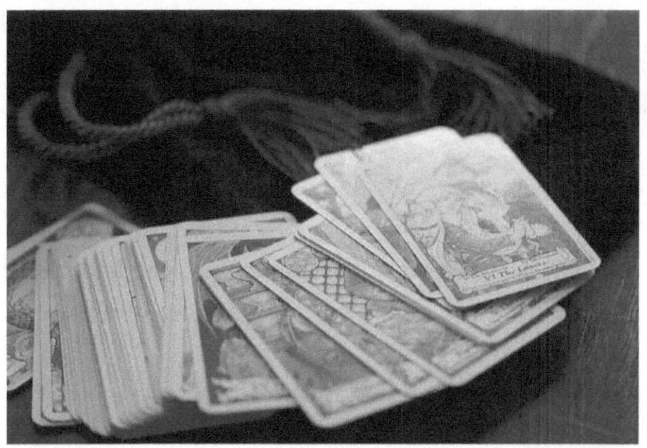

But what exactly is a psychic? Have you ever had the feeling that someone is going to call you or been thinking of a person and shortly after run into them? Or have you ever dreamt of things that later happen in reality? Do you have constant déjà vu experiences? These are typical signs of psychic abilities. The vast majority of people have psychic abilities in a certain form or shape, and it is most commonly a guardian, a parent, or an adult that will first notice the signs of psychic behavior. Unfortunately, there are some people that think of psychics as evil and that they practice black magic, something that is simply not true. We all depict some sort of psychic behavior but many of us do not know how to acknowledge the symptoms or we simply ignore them because we do not know them yet. Let us see some signs that indicate you are in possession of psychic abilities:

- Higher intuition levels:

For instance, knowing who is calling you before you even pick up the phone or knowing you are going to receive a text before your phone rings. Predicting things before they even happen means that you have a higher level of intuition.

- Experiencing déjà vu countless times:

Getting the feeling that you have already been somewhere even though you haven't, or you feel extremely at ease and familiar with places, things, and people you most probably experience déjà vu. This experience is a certain sign that you have a type of psychic ability.

• Visions are something normal for you:

In case you are having visions of future events you have psychic abilities even if they are expressed in dreams or when you are awake.

• Your gut feeling is always accurate:

If you simply know that something is going to happen before it does and you are able to sense events that are currently happening or are about to happen, you have a strong sign that you are a psychic.

• Telepathic instances:

Do you feel as if you are able to send messages to others using your mind? Do you think that you are reading the thoughts of others? Have you ever experienced a connection to someone else's mind? If you have, then you have some form of telepathy which is a sign that you are a psychic.

• Premonitions and Predictions:

Have you ever seen events that you simply know they will happen sometime in the future? Have they actually happened? If you told someone about them or wrote them down before they happened and then they did, you have one of the psychic gifts.

• Psychometry is evident:

Psychometry is the ability of psychics to allow a person to experience or sense the story of an object or person by only touching them. Psychics have such power and knowledge because they know and are aware of energies, places, objects, and people simply by touching someone or something. For instance, a psychic that has this ability can touch a person's hand and experience as well as sense their past.

- Vivid and powerful dreams:

People that are gifted with psychic abilities have very vivid dreams and are able to remember the smallest detail after they awake. They know that the symbols they see in their dreams have deep-rooted meanings and are essential to understand life experiences.

- You can sense trouble:

This is a strong feeling and occurs when you know that someone you love is in trouble. It has a great impact on your psychology and is often accompanied by a strong sense of fear. There is no other explanation for it aside from the fact that you know something is seriously wrong with the person you love.

- You can tell the future:

This is one of the most common traits when it comes to psychic abilities. Letting your family and friends know about the future and then actually happening is a sure sign that you are a psychic.

- You can heal:

Have you ever experienced getting your hands on someone who is ill or suffering? Have you seen a change for the better in this person? Many who have psychic abilities can heal others by using their energy.

- Hearing sounds:

Did you ever hear sounds that other people in your presence could not? Are you wondering constantly why no one can hear chimes and beeps? Such sounds can indicate an event that is going to happen in the near future and can warn you about particular events that are about to occur.

- You can sense two places at the same time:

This is one of the strongest abilities that psychics have. For example, you may be home or at a place you are comfortable and sense experiences and events happening in different places. Then, you are most probably a psychic. If you have visions of events that actually happen, and you feel as if you are transported to this destination your abilities are also heightened.

Your psychic abilities are not something that should scare you or be afraid of. You should treasure these gifts and unique skills as well as learn more about each ability so as to awaken them and develop to their full potential. Many of such skills are very helpful for those who have not yet discovered their own gifts since people often turn to psychics for different reasons but mostly for support and guidance.

Below you will find a list of the known psychic abilities:

- Astral projection: the ability to voluntarily separate the astral body.
- Apportation: the ability to conduct the teleportation, disappearance, or materialization of an object.
- Automatic writing: the ability to write or draw without consciously intending to.
- Dowsing: the ability to locate water.
- Divination: the ability to have insight into an event using occult means.
- Energy medicine: the ability to heal with your own astral, spiritual, mental, empathic, or etheric energy.
- Mediumship or channeling: the ability to contact spirits.
- Levitation: the ability to fly or float by mystical ways.
- Precognition: the ability to see future events.
- Psychokinesis: the ability to manipulate objects with your mind.

- Psychic surgery: the ability to eliminate a disorder or disease within the body through energetic incision.
- Psychometry: the ability to gain information about an object or a person by touch.
- Telepathy: the ability to transmit thoughts supernaturally.
- Retrocognition: the ability to perceive past events.

Most of the people in the metaphysical world believe that all of us are born with different degrees of intuition. However, as children, we learn to develop our rational left part of the brain, completely ignoring the more creative, intuitive, and spiritual right side of the brain. As a result, many people out of fear suppress their psychic abilities and bury such gifts leaving them dormant for the rest of their lives. There are a lot of things to gain by awakening and developing these abilities for both yourself and others. We all are spiritual beings that continue to evolve in many positive ways.

According to Hereward Carrington, metaphysician and author of the book "Your Psychic Powers and How To Develop Them":

"It all depends on which channel we direct the energy of our will. The soul must learn to find and experience itself fully before it can consider itself thoroughly alive and a fully developed entity. After this realization has been accomplished, then, and then only, should we direct our attention to cultivating and directing the latent energies which we possess."

The first thing you can do to awaken and develop your psychic abilities is to meditate. Any form of meditation will benefit your spiritual, physical, and emotional health. Meditation has been proven to lower your stress levels, blood pressure, and gain peace of mind. There have been incidents of people who report that they have trouble meditating and the truth is that they are making this process more complicated than it really is. Meditation is much easier for everybody if they start practicing it in its simplest forms first.

It is believed that while prayer is the way to talk to God, meditation is the way to listen to God. However, do not confuse meditation with religion. Even though meditation has been practiced in most religions for thousands of years, it is not a belief system or a doctrine. If you set a particular time to meditate and do it regularly, then you will be directing your energy to your higher self. This practice of meditation will meld over time your conscious and spiritual mind. It will transform you for the better. Your energy will clear and your senses will be enhanced as you will slowly but steadily gain awareness of the psychic realm.

Transcendental meditation is recommended for this case since it is a great way to focus on your spiritual energy and clear your mind. Start by meditating on a daily basis for seven to ten minutes each day. After a week passes, you can start meditating for 15 minutes each day. Over the past decade, this type of meditation has turned out to be very popular. Transcendental meditation is a form of a mantra meditation introduced to the Western culture in 1950 by Maharishi Mahesh Yogi. He was the one that taught this meditation type all over the world for about 40 years.

All that is needed to practice this form of meditation is to sit somewhere comfortable with your eyes closed. You don't need a certain posture or pose, you just need to be alone and in a quiet room with a comfortable chair that will help you start the practice, and once you are familiar with this meditation technique you can practice it anywhere. The only thing that you need to do is to keep your eyes closed and chant silently your mantra. A mantra essentially is a meaningless sound with no real secrets behind it except that it should sound positive.

There is no point losing time to choose the perfect mantra since the less you know about the mantra you are using the better it will be for your practice. The most common mantra is *Om*. However, most teachers do not use this mantra due to the wholeness of the sound it makes. According to Hinduism, this sound reflects all the combined vibrations both negative and positive. This mantra is mostly practiced by monks. Other mantras include:

- *Aema*
- *Inga*
- *Kirim*
- *Shirim*

It would be preferable to not try different mantras during your meditation practice. According to most teachers, their students use the same mantra they did on their first meditation practice because the aim is not to find the right sound.

Breathing is also very important to slow down your mind to develop your psychic skills. It is not possible to have a psychic connection when you are in a common state of consciousness. Through breathing, you will slow your body to reach a relaxed state of mind that will allow you to form a connection with your abilities. While you breathe, you will instantly notice all the things you have not seen before. You will feel and hear yourself breathe; you will be living directly in the moment. While you are meditating, you will become extremely aware of the patterns and sounds in nature, both your emotions and your physical environment. Through this enhanced awareness, understanding and insight most commonly come to surface.

If you maintain an attitude of the person who wishes to understand, you will start seeing life in a whole new way. However, you should not keep this attitude only during meditation but you should also have it throughout your everyday life too. As you expand your awareness, you will develop the intention to receive information through your emotions, mind, and body. Everything is connected to the universe and as your psychic awareness develops, you will start to feel, hear, and see all such connections.

You should not rush and get frustrated when you are trying to awaken and develop your psychic abilities. Intuition and psychic powers are not developed instantly. Every skill that you learn takes time and effort to be fully developed and still there is always something new to learn about it. Every person develops at his or her own rate. If you are consistent then your sixth sense will grow with daily meditation and the practice of awareness being key to how you will progress. Keep practicing directing your energy towards answers and solutions.

You need to be open in learning and growing your abilities so as to grab any opportunity that will present itself. There is no reason to try to awaken and develop your psychic abilities on your own. Attend lectures, seminars, guided meditations, and get connected with your local metaphysical community. If you are having trouble with meditation, you can get a wide variety of books, tapes, or search for other resources that will help you. Search articles, blogs, forums, and educational sites that will offer you valuable information. However, you should also find people that have already developed and awakened their psychic abilities. They are the most informed and knowledgeable on the subject that will help you the most.

Keep track of your progress so as to know where you are at. Write down your impressions and your dreams with as much detail as you can. If you encounter repeating symbols and details in your Third Eye, they are important. Try to use your newfound insights and knowledge by writing them down and trying to explain them.

Awakening and developing your psychic abilities is a personal decision but know that spiritual growth will be the result of a positive decision. You will open windows and doors that you may not have understood in the past and when combined with an awakened and balanced Third Eye, your psychic abilities will offer you deep and profound knowledge about different worlds. You will open yourself to receive messages that hold a wisdom not many people are lucky to have and use it for the greater good. Ignore what others may think about your path and trust your first instinct. Practice makes perfect and for this reason, you should be gentle with yourself if you do not see immediate results. Your psychic abilities need time to be awakened and developed as it the case with your Third Eye, however, when they do awaken, the benefits you will receive will have been worth your time. You give to yourself a valuable gift, access to your soul, and be certain that your soul will never let you down.

HOW TO SEAL THE AURA

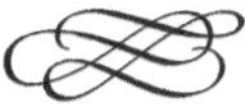

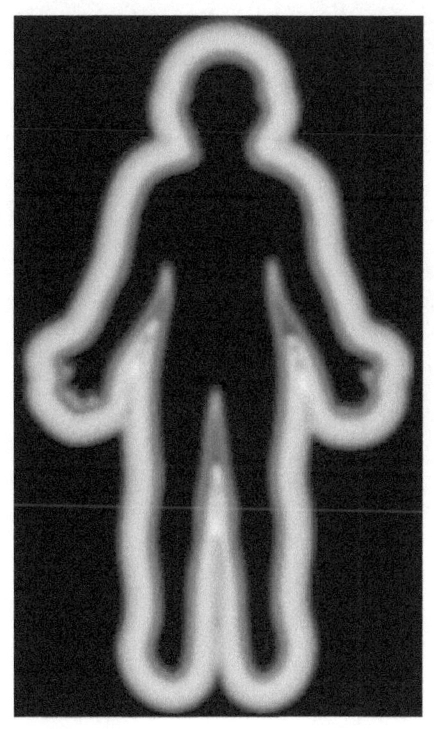

You must have heard about the aura, the electromagnetic energy field that surrounds the body. Well, have you ever come across a person who made you feel nervous without a particular reason? Or meeting a person that made you feel completely comfortable in his or her presence? In such moments, you are having a reaction to the energy of a person. On an energetic level, our auras, are connected with our chakras as well as our overall state of consciousness.

In esoteric traditions, the subtle body is indicated as the aura while holistic medicine practitioners and psychics claim to be able to see the color, type of vibration, and the size of an aura. In spiritual alternative medicine, the aura of humans is believed to be part of a hidden anatomy that represents the state of health of the client and it is even believed that includes the viral force of the chakras. However, such theories are not supported by science and are labeled as pseudo-science.

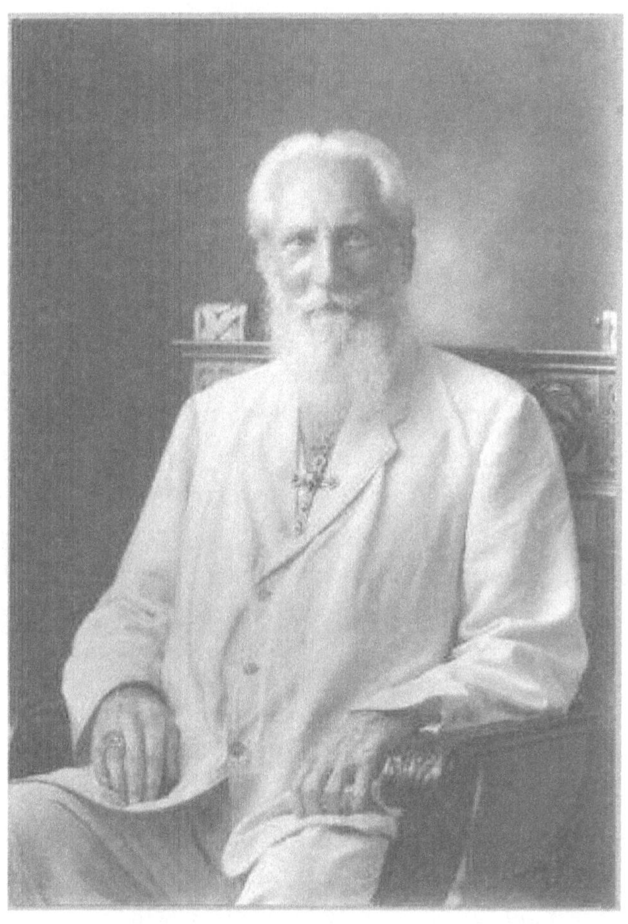

The idea of auras first became popular by Charles Webster Leadbeater who was a member of the mystic Theosophical Society and a former priest of the Church of England. He had studied theosophy in India, and he wanted to use his clairvoyant powers to conduct scientific investigations. Leadbeater claimed that most men come from Mars and the more advanced men come from the Moon. Also, he claimed that hydrogen atoms are constructed of six bodies included in and form similar to an egg. His book "Man Visible and Invisible" published in 1903, depicted the human aura at different stages of the moral evolution that ranged from savage to saint.

Later, in 1910, he presented the modern concept of auras in his book

"The Inner Life" by including the Tantric notion of chakras. However, he didn't only show the Tantric beliefs in the Western civilization but reinterpreted and reconstructed them with a mix of his own ideas without giving acknowledgments to the sources of such innovations. The attempts to capture the energy field that surrounds the human body date back many years and more specifically to the French physician, Hippolyte Baraduc, in the 1890s.

These images have received supernatural interpretations that have been the result of a lack of understanding of the natural phenomena associated with them such as the emanating heat from the human body that produces images similar to aura under infrared photography. Semyon Davidovich Kirlian discovered in 1939 that when he placed a body part or an object directly on photographic paper and passed a high voltage across that body part or object, he was able to get an image of a glowing contour surrounding the object. This process became what was later known as Kirlian photography.

According to various parapsychologists at such as Thelma Moss of UCLA, such images depict the levels of bioenergies and psychic powers. However, various studies have discovered that the Kirlian effects happened due to the presence of moisture on an object when it is being photographed. Electricity produces an area of gas ionization in the area around the object when it is moist which is what happens to all living things. This will alter the electric charge pattern on the film and after repeated experiments, no hidden process has been discovered when it comes to Kirlian photography.

However, the consensus in the scientific community is that everything in the world produces a certain type of energy, so despite the fact that the existence of auras has not been proven yet it is not a ludicrous concept. To auras, there are seven layers which are also known as the subtle bodies and correspond with the seven chakras in your body. The first one is the physical aura layer that diminishes during waking hours and rejuvenates throughout our sleep. It is connected to our overall bodily health and five senses. You can see this layer named the etheric layer also and is the closest one to our physical body.

The second one is the astral aura layer or else the emotional layer and is connected to our emotions. This is the layer that stores emotional experiences and memories. It extends three inches away from our bodies. The lower aura layer or the mental layer is connected to the way we think and to logic. This is the layer where we spend most of our waking hours. It is active when we work, study, or focus on the various tasks we have during the day. This layer is away from our body by three to eight inches and is also related to our ego, beliefs, and values.

The higher aura layer or else the astral body is the higher layer that connects the wellbeing of others to your wellbeing. It is the place where our self-compassion and selflessness are produced. Otherwise known as the love layer, it is connected with the heart chakra and sits at the middle of the seven chakra system so it is believed to link the three lower auric planes with the higher ones. The spiritual aura layer or else the manifestation layer, or the etheric double, is able to connect you with other people over spiritual matters. Your aura will shine and grow brighter when you share, engage, and teach with others on a spiritual level.

The intuitional aura layer or the celestial plane is the sixth aura layer which essentially is your Third Eye, it will allow you to achieve a deeper level of awareness and your intuition as well as your sensitivity is heightened. In the end, there is the absolute aura layer, or else the ketheric template, or the "I Am" layer, which depicts your connection with the divine and stores your every experience as well as guides you in your path in life.

Each of the aura levels is believed to be portrayed by a different color. The color of your aura shows how spiritually, physically, and mentally dynamic you are. For example, some levels may be duller when you are sick or sad while others could be brighter where you have vibrant energy. Energy practitioners and spiritual advisors have offered general interpretations of the meaning of the aura color. Some of them are:

- Green: you feel connected to nature, healers. This is a calming and comfortable color. People with green auras enjoy helping others and are peaceful as well as compassionate.
- Turquoise: natural organizer, dynamic personality.
- Purple: you are a spiritual and sensitive person. A person with a purple aura may have heightened psychic abilities.
- Pink: you are peaceful and harmonious. Pink auras are rare and indicate that you are kind, loving, and gentle.
- Red: you are vibrant and passionate. This is the color filled with passion and energy. It is related to material goods, the earth, and the physical body.
- Yellow: you are intellectual and joyful. This color is often associated with psychic and spiritual awakening as well as with intellect, optimism, and with happiness.
- White: you are in harmony and balanced.
- Blue: you are intuitive and spiritual. The traits associated with this color are seriousness, authority, and calmness.
- Murky: you are physically or mentally ill.
- Orange: it means that you are ambitious or creative. You express your emotions and you are outgoing.

As you can see, certain colors point out your strengths while others signal problems such as muddy colors like gray or brown which can indicate depression or other ailments. If your aura is mostly white it can be an indication that there is a lack of harmony between your body and your mind. For instance, you will see a mostly white aura in people who are in a near-death state due to the fact that there is a growing separation between the mind and the body. Before you start working with your aura or attempt to read the auras of other people, you will first need to know how to recognize it. There are many who have an innate ability to sense and see them, but there are also many that need to practice to be able to do so.

An easy way to practice is to look at your reflection in the mirror with a neutral or white background. Do this at a time where you will have no distractions or interruptions for at least a few minutes. Feel your eyes relax and eventually, you will witness a soft white light that surrounds you. Maintain your focus for a bit more and you will start seeing colors. You can also practice sensing your aura too. Again, be at a place where you will not be disturbed and place yourself in a comfortable position. Have the palms of your hands approximately six inches away from your body. Maintain that distance and move your hands up and down all over your body. Do it in slow movements to give yourself time to sense the colors and feel the impressions you are getting. It can also help sometimes to rapidly rub your hands together before you do this exercise to open the sensitivity in the minor chakras located on your hands.

Empaths and highly sensitive people may be able to read auras quicker than other people, but the truth is that anyone can learn how to see auras because we all have an inner psychic. It only needs determination and practice to achieve this amazing skill. You can start by paying attention to the emotions and energy of other people when you are in their presence. It is admittedly easier to sense the energy before you start visualizing it. Be aware of both your emotions and those of others. How do you think they feel? How do they make you feel? How do you instinctively respond to their emotions? It would be best to start with a person you know well and not with a stranger since you will already be familiar with their moods and behavior. As you practice and your confidence in your abilities grows, you can do this to someone you do not know very well.

It is a fact that the auras of humans are the most difficult and complex to see. So, it would be best to start with something simpler such as reading the aura of a plant, a popular choice for beginners. They have stronger auras than inanimate objects, however, they are easy to read. Stare at a particular spot of a plant for at least 30 seconds. Keep your eyes focused on that particular spot and let your gaze soften and go slightly unfocused as if you are trying to see through the plant. Extend your vision further out to look at the periphery. This is the time when you will start noticing the aura that surrounds the plant.

If you find the above practices difficult, place a plant at the front of a neutral background such as a white wall that will provide the necessary contrast and as a result make the colors of the plant's aura easier to notice. Once you have mastered reading the aura of plants you chose, you can move on to other plants or objects with bright colors. It is important to do your best and create a relaxing environment. For this reason, you will need lighting that is not too soft or too harsh. You can even listen to relaxing music to create the right atmosphere. Also, you could meditate beforehand to be focused and relaxed as you practice.

When you are ready to practice on a person, you should start with a friend that you trust and always ask their permission first. It is important for you to have the other person's consent. Position your friend against a neutral background and stand approximately 12 to 18 inches away from them. Apply the same method we showed you above with the plant. As you focus your gaze, you can use any of your senses to feel the colors of the aura and not only your vision. Once you have successfully made a connection, you can ask of your friend for him or her to move around and see if you can still feel the same colors.

As is the case with most skills in life practice makes perfect. So, you need to keep practicing in order to read and see auras as well as to improve your abilities. Keep practicing with family and friends and do not be afraid to try and read your own aura too. You are the one who knows you better than anyone else, so it will be easier for you to read your own aura than that of another person. One of the main purposes of the aura is to act as a protective shield between us and other living beings. If it wasn't for the aura we would be on the receiving end of others' spiritual, mental, and emotional states all the time which may be what we wish to achieve in intuitive practices but only when we are able to control it and safeguard ourselves. There are several signs of a defective aura and having your aura operate and be effectively sealed is extremely important since there should be no rents or rifts. Some of the symptoms are:

- Poor boundaries.
- Headaches.

- Uncontrollable emotions such as anxiety fear or paranoia.
- Feelings of isolation.
- Lack of personal space.

Damage to your aura is usually caused by:

- Mental or emotional difficulties such as anger and stress.
- Psychic attack – someone wishing you ill.
- Poor health.
- Poor auric hygiene.
- Invasive surgery.
- Alcohol and drug addictions.
- Accidents or events that cause shock.

The first thing you can do to seal your aura is basic self-care such as eating good, resting, and make sure you exercise. Then, you should work to eliminate any lingering negativity. Even though life is not always blissful or easy, focusing solely on your negative thoughts is never good for you in the long run. Do your best to take time out of your schedule and appreciate the beauty that exists around you. For instance, place fresh flowers in a vase, appreciate the smell of a warm cup of coffee, the smile of your loved ones, and the sunset. Make sure that you add some beauty in your home and in your surroundings.

Practicing meditation can also help you seal and clean your aura since it brings your spirit, mind, and body back into balance. As we will see in the following chapter, meditation can be practiced anywhere and even a few minutes a day can make you see a very strong difference in yourself. It is an amazing tool for emotional healing and will allow you to stay aware and present as you deal with obstacles that cross your path. Using the positive affirmations, we mentioned in the previous chapter can also help in washing away the stress of the day. Affirmations work their way into the subconscious and conscious mind to help us reprogram our belief systems that limit us. By repeating positive affirmations, you will replace your negative thoughts and your newly formed positive mindset will become a part of who you are.

Always remember that everything is energy and we are made of energy too. Our energy can be affected by many factors and is very sensitive. With auras you will always know what your energetic state at any time and any place is. No one can deny that the body and the mind are closely connected and the aura is believed to represent this link. Learning more things about your aura such as how to seal it and cleanse it and finding out how to read the auras of others can take time. So, be patient and keep practicing because it is very helpful to know how to be aware of your energy and how it affects the people that surround you.

HEALING MEDITATION

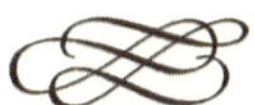

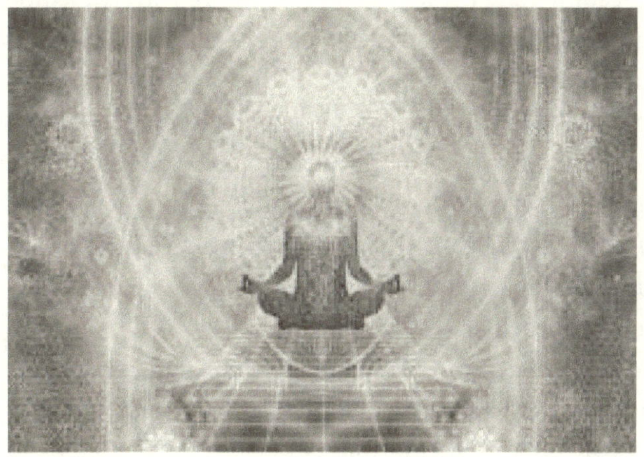

The practice of focusing and thinking deeply for a certain period of time, or else meditation, is found deeply rooted in ancient civilizations and practiced by cultures and religions from all over the world. The earliest evidence for the existence of meditation that we have, are wall arts from the Indus Valley dated around 5,000 and 3,500 BCE. They illustrate people resting on the ground with their hands on their knees and their legs crossed, a position that is widely recognized as the most famous one of meditation practice.

Ancient Indian scriptures have offered us meditation techniques of over 3,000 years ago. Nowadays, meditation is not practiced only for religious purposes but is primarily used as the main tool of many to calm their mind and bring forth feelings of peace and relaxation. There are several types of meditation since it is practiced in various forms and if you are a beginner that wishes to enjoy the benefits of meditation, below you will find a list of the most common meditation types:

- Transcendental Meditation: This is a simple meditation technique where a personally assigned mantra, most commonly a familiar and calming word or a phrase, is repeated in a particular way.
- Mindfulness Meditation: This is the process through which you become fully present and in harmony with your thoughts without concerning yourself with everything that goes on around you.
- Mantra Meditation: This meditation technique also uses a mantra, a calming word or phrase, to help the person from having distracting thoughts when meditating.
- *Vipassana* Meditation: This is an ancient Indian form of meditation where you see things as they really are - the meaning of the Sanskrit word *Vipassana*.
- Guided Meditation: This is a method through which you visualize situations or mental pictures that relax you.
- Loving-Kindness Meditation: Otherwise known as *Metta* meditation, this practice will have you direct your kind wishes upon others.
- Yoga Meditation: This is another ancient Indian practice through which you perform a number of postures along with breathing control exercises that aim to promote the calm of the mind and flexibility.
- Chakra Meditation: This is a set of relaxation exercises that focus on healing and bringing balance to your chakras as well as spiritual power to your body.

Meditation has many benefits that are widely accepted even by the scientific community. For instance, when regularly practicing meditation, you will find a significant stress reduction which is actually one of the most common reasons people start to meditate in the first place. Usually, physical and mental stress lead to increased levels of cortisol, the stress hormone. As a result, this hormone causes the various harmful effects of stress such as disruption of sleep, anxiety, depression, increased blood pressure, and fatigue.

Meditation can also help you control anxiety since less stress translates to less anxiety. It has also helped lessen symptoms of various anxiety disorders such as social anxiety, phobias, paranoid thoughts, panic attacks, and obsessive-compulsive behaviors. Emotional health can also be maintained at its optimal level with some forms of meditation that can lead to a more positive outlook on life and improved self-confidence and self-image. Mindfulness meditation is often recommended for such cases of people who wish to develop and maintain their emotional health.

Enhanced self-awareness is another benefit you will experience by practicing meditation often since it can help you understand yourself better as well as help you grow into your best self. For instance, self-inquiry meditation will help you not only understand yourself better but also how you are related to the people around you. There are other forms of meditation that help you recognize the various thoughts that may be self-defeating and harmful by gaining awareness of the habit of your thoughts. When your thoughts start to become negative, you will learn how to direct them towards more constructive paths.

People who meditate by practicing focused-attention meditation have reported that they have successfully lengthened their attention span. This form of meditation exercises your attention span and makes it stronger by increasing the endurance of your attention. Even meditating for a short while can be very beneficial for you so as to grow your attention span. For instance, one study discovered that four days of such meditation is enough.

There have also been reports that meditation may reduce memory loss that comes with age. As we have mentioned, meditation improves our clarity of thinking and attention, two factors that may help keep the mind still young despite physical age. A method of meditation named *Kirtan Kriya* combines a chant or a mantra along with the repetitive motion of the fingers so as to focus thoughts. Meditation has also shown promising results for partially improving memory-related issues especially for patients with dementia.

Kindness is certainly something that can be learned through meditation since several types of meditation increase positive actions towards others and yourself as well as positive feelings. For example, the loving-kindness meditation or *Metta* we previously mentioned, starts with your developing kind feelings and thoughts towards yourself. As you keep practicing, you learn how to expand this forgiveness and kindness to first friends, acquaintances, and at the end, even to enemies.

Meditation is even recommended to people who suffer from addictive behaviors. This is the case because to complete a meditation practice you need to develop your mental discipline and as a result, it can help you break dependencies by increasing your awareness, your self-control and help you understand what truly triggers such addictive behaviors. According to research, meditation can help many people to understand how to redirect their focus, increase their willpower, understand the causes of their addictive behaviors, and control their impulses, including food cravings, as well as their emotions.

There are many people who suffer or will suffer from insomnia at some point in their lives. Mindfulness meditation can help in sleep improvement by redirecting your prolific thoughts that are often the cause of insomnia. It will help you relax your body and place you in a peaceful state by releasing tension. As a result, you are more likely to fall asleep. Similarly, meditation helps control the pain since our perception of pain is linked to our state of mind which can be enhanced when we go through stressful situations. With meditation, you will feel still feel pain, but you will develop the enhanced ability to cope with it and maybe even experience a reduced sensation of pain.

All these meditation benefits are backed by science and are not only worth your time spend on meditating, but it should also prompt you to start meditating. As you can see from the benefits listed above, meditation evidently can help you overcome illnesses. Healing meditation which is also known as mindfulness practice is a practice that aims to exercise your mental relaxation and focus. The term mindfulness is a technique designed and used for thousands of years and is also known as transcendental meditation. Its origins can be traced in India and more specifically in the *Vedic* tradition. It is strongly connected with the yoga system and with *Ayurvedic* medicine. Principles of meditation can be traced in *Qigong, Tai Chi*, breath regulation, and the relaxation response.

For many years, meditation was believed to be the way to solve all life's problems. However, it is more the ability to experience a peaceful mind but even this is a small part of the meditation practice and many people are not able to achieve this with only a simple daily practice. This particular misconception left meditation on the sidelines for a long time since it was not able to solve everything as many believed. However, today, meditation is practiced by millions with a clear intent that it has profound health benefits. Mindfulness can be simply put as if noticing what happens to each moment in life no matter if the events are difficult, painful, easy, or joyful.

The powers of healing meditation have been studied and debated by many scientists because it is not clearly understood how it has such amazing results on the health benefits concerning the body. We already know that shifting our mindset has powerful benefits. For instance, the placebo effect has shown us its healing capabilities without even the use of medicine or a drug. The only thing it did is to establish the belief that there was an intervention. One of the various studies on the placebo effect used a group and instructed them to receive a pill with an active ingredient whilst another group was given a sugar pill. Both groups did not know which pill they were given. The placebo was discovered to have measured various benefits to those who believed that they have in treated while they only received a sugar pill. This phenomenon has baffled researchers and it can be explained by the fact that the brain is a very complex organ and meditation apparently has many benefits when it comes to healing.

Neuroscience started to measure how meditation benefits the human brain. One study researched brain activity with magnetic resonance (MR) before and after a meditation practice and within a timeframe of eight weeks. The University of Massachusetts found in the study, "Mindfulness practice leads to increases in regional brain gray matter density," by Britta K.Hölzelab James Carmody MarkVangel, Christina Congleton, Sita M.Yerramsettia, TimGard, and Sara W.Lazara this:

- The analysis of the images located a decrease in grey matter density in the brain.
- More specifically, they measured various changes in the hippocampus, which is believed to be important for memory and learning as well as it being associated with introspection, compassion, and self-awareness.
- They also found in the images a decrease in the density in other parts of the brain.
- The amygdala which plays an essential role in stress and anxiety had a decrease in grey matter.

Studies have also been conducted for the long-term effects healing meditation has on the brain. A study conducted in 2012: "Effects of mindful-attention and compassion meditation training on amygdala response to emotional stimuli in an ordinary, non-meditative state," by Gaëlle Desbordes, Lobsang T. Negi, Thaddeus W. W. Pace, B. Alan Wallace, Charles L. Raison, and Eric L. Schwartz, used functional magnetic resonance imaging (fMRI) to test exactly this. The researchers found:

- Changes in the brain activation in the amygdala.

- Changes in brain activity in people that remained even when they were not meditating.

The conclusion was that meditation can induce learning that is not specific to tasks but process-specific in the brain. This can result in enduring changes in mental function. However, the strongest evidence of healing meditation shown in various studies is for the treatment of depression and anxiety. Why? Meditating for a long term can have long term benefits on the ability and performance of the human brain. A study was conducted with the participation of Tibetan Buddhist monks: "Long-term meditators self-induce high-amplitude gamma synchrony during mental practice" by Antoine Lutz, Lawrence L. Greischar, Nancy B. Rawlings, Matthieu Ricard, and Richard J. Davidson, and it was discovered that they showed an increase in gamma activity in the brain. More specifically,

- Meditation can potentially increase the number of gamma waves in the brain which are the smallest kinds of energy in the brain and are linked with feelings of blessing.
- The monks demonstrated a huge increase in gamma rays not previously seen before.

Other studies, such as the "Hemodynamic responses on prefrontal cortex related to meditation and attentional task" by Singh Deepeshwar, Suhas Ashok Vinchurkar, Naveen Kalkuni Visweswaraiah, and Hongasandra RamaRao Nagendra, have shown that the long term practice of meditation and similar attention training can increase the thickness as well as the blood flow to the prefrontal cortex which is the area linked with decision making, shaping personality, and complex behavior. For high performing people this is an essential functional area of the brain.

However, healing meditation extends beyond the function and the structure of the brain. Research in the 1970s, "A wakeful hypometabolic physiologic state" by RK Wallace, H Benson, and AF Wilson, discovered that meditation can change the way our body works. For instance, mindfulness can induce a 'hypo-metabolic' state, something similar to hibernation. By achieving this state, its benefits include the help of healing and prolonging the life of the cells in our bodies. The consumption of oxygen decreases, resulting in it entering a relaxed state.

Nowadays our insight into the human gut microbiome has helped us understand how this state happens. Trillions of microbes reside in the digestive system and manage the gut lining and immune system. It is a fact that stress can greatly affect gut microbes. Meditation can aid us in regulating the gut microbes stress response by the replacement of chronic inflammation states and maintenance of a healthy gut barrier function. The gut microbe can not only affect the immune system but also the expression of DNA genes. Based on various studies such as "What Is the Molecular Signature of Mind-Body Interventions? A Systematic Review of Gene Expression Changes Induced by Meditation and Related Practices" by Ivana Buric, Miguel Farias, Jonathan Jong, Christopher Mee, and Inti A. Brazil, meditation can regulate pro-inflammatory genes that in turn regulate inflammation. The effects move through the brain and these genes were discovered to increase the response time of the brain to the cortisol stress hormone when they were challenged with mental calculations and speech in front of an audience.

Conditions such as Type 2 diabetes, Alzheimer's disease, and inflammatory digestive conditions are connected to intestinal permeability. When stress hormones are reduced such as epinephrine and cortisol through relaxation and rest as well as meditation and mindful eating, these tight junctions can heal. The majority of the neurotransmitters in the body are released through the gut microbiome. With meditation, we can help ourselves in regulating the stress response and suppress chronic inflammation as well as have a healthy gut barrier function.

The connection between the brain and the gut is an essential factor when we are dealing with a chronic digestive disorder. For this reason, healing meditation for digestive diseases is supported by various studies such as "Meditation and vacation effects have an impact on disease-associated molecular phenotypes" by E S Epel, E Puterman, J Lin, E H Blackburn, P Y Lum, N D Beckmann, J Zhu, E Lee, A Gilbert, R A Rissman, R E Tanzi, and E E Schadt. In this study, it was discovered that stress management methods, as well as other psychological techniques, can help people with irritable bowel syndrome. The results were very promising for at least the short term.

Based on research, chronic inflammation can cause many chronic diseases. A set of genes are activated in the body through chronic inflammation. Intestinal permeability or a leaky gut are connected to many auto-immune, digestive, and metabolic disorders which are all linked with inflammation. The study "What Is the Molecular Signature of Mind-Body Interventions? A Systematic Review of Gene Expression Changes Induced by Meditation and Related Practices" by Ivana Buric, Miguel Farias, Jonathan Jong, Christopher Mee, and Inti A. Brazil, has concluded that mindfulness can help in the production of the opposite gene activation as it happens with inflammation.

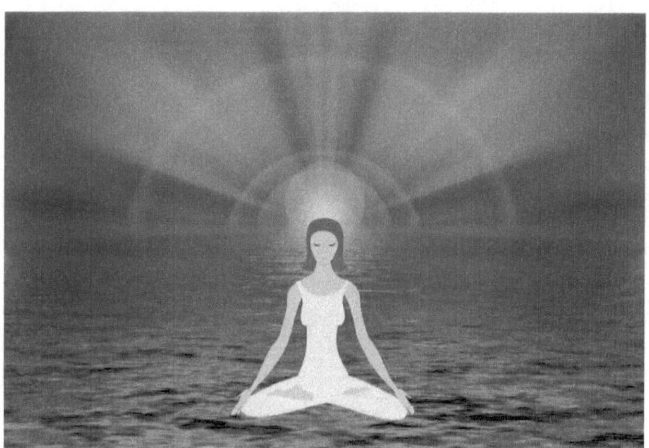

But why is mindfulness or healing meditation so effective? Mindfulness meditation is essentially teaching you how to slow down any racing thoughts, both in your body and your mind and let go of negativity. Generally, mindfulness practices vary but almost every one includes awareness of mind and body as well as everything practice.

With mindfulness meditation, you don't need essential oils, mantras, or candles, unless you wish to include them in your practice. To start practicing mindfulness meditation all you need is three or five minutes of your time to free your mind of judgments, and a comfortable place to sit.

Teaching yourself mindfulness meditation is very straightforward but if you are at a beginner level, a program or teacher will help you greatly to get started, especially if you're practicing this meditation type for health reasons. Make sure that you always have time for yourself to practice mindfulness meditation even if you have to set your alarm half an hour earlier than normal in the morning but do not be very hard on yourself since life gets in the way sometimes, just try again tomorrow.

The first step when it comes to meditation is to find a comfortable and quiet place to practice. You can either sit on the floor or in a chair with your back, head and neck straight but not stiff. It will also help if you wear loose, comfortable clothing so as to not be distracted. Even though it is not necessary, you can use a timer or a gentle and soft alarm to help you forget about time and focus on your medication as well as strip you of excuses for stopping and doing something else.

Many people lose track of time while they meditate and a timer or an alarm will make it certain that you are not meditating for very long. After you finish your meditation session allow yourself some time to get up gradually and become aware of where you are. Be aware of your breath and be in tune with the sensation of the moving air in and out of your body as you breathe. Be aware of your belly falling and rising as the air enters your nostrils and leaves your mouth. Focus your attention because each breath is different, and it changes. If you notice thoughts entering your mind do not suppress them or ignore them. Remain calm and acknowledge them by using your breath as a guide.

However, if you see that your thoughts persist whether due to anxiety, hope, fear, or worry, observe where your mind takes you without judging yourself and simply return your focus to breathing.

There is no reason to judge yourself when this happens because the practice of refocusing on your breath and on the present is practicing mindfulness. Let us see the steps of a full mindfulness meditation practice:

- Take a seat wherever you feel comfortable. Find a spot that offers you a solid and stable seat that will not have you hanging back.
- If you are on the floor on a cushion, cross your legs in front of you in a way that will still keep you comfortable. If you are on a chair, it would be good for the bottom of your feet to touch the floor.
- Do not stiffen your upper body, just keep it straight. The spine has a natural curvature, do not suppress it.
- Place your upper arms in a parallel manner to your upper body and then, let your hands fall at the top of your legs. As you have your upper arms at your sides, your hands will be in the right spot.
- Drop your chin and let your eyes fall softly forward. If you feel like it, you can have your eyelids fall completely closed but while meditating it is not essential to close your eyes.
- Stay there for a few moments and simply relax. Focus your attention on the sensations in your body or to your breath.
- Feel your breath and the sensations it causes as to moves inside and then outside of your body. Focus on the sensation of breathing.
- Inevitably, especially for beginners, your focus will be shifted from your breath and move on to other places. There is no need to worry about that since you can turn gently your attention back to your breath.
- Before you move your body in any way, practice pausing. For instance, if you wish to scratch an itch, shift with intention at a moment of your choosing to allow some space between what you experience and what you choose to do.
- When you finish your session, lift your gaze gently and open your eyes. Give yourself some time to notice and be aware of

your environment. Be aware of how your body feels at this specific moment. Be aware of your emotions and thoughts.

You can also practice mindfulness meditation in your everyday life since you can do most things in a mindful way. According to Megan Monahan, the author of "Don't Hate, Meditate" – "Anytime that you are resting your attention in the present moment and whatever you are doing/experiencing you are practicing being mindful. Not only does this enrich the present moment activity/experience you're engaging in, but it also allows you to be present in your time rather than going back into the past or the future".

Some ways that you can start practicing mindfulness in everyday life are:

- Driving: Do not turn the radio on and if you do put on something relaxing such as classical music. Visualize your spine growing tall by finding the point half-way between gripping the wheel too tightly and relaxing your hands. As you feel your mind wandering, bring it back to where you and your car are in space.
- Brushing your teeth: Focus on your feet touching the floor, the movement of your arm, and the brush in your hand.
- Doing the dishes: Relish the feeling of warm water on your hands and focus on the bubbles and the sounds the dishes are making.
- Exercising: Opt to focus on your breathing instead of watching television as well as on the movement of your feet as you walk.
- Doing laundry: Focus your attention on the scent of clean clothes and the soft feel of the fabric.
- Preparing kids for bed: Get on the same level as your kids, listen more, look in their eyes, and relish in their snuggles. When you are relaxed, they will also be relaxed.

Many people often give up on the greatness of healing meditation because they expect too much too soon. The truth is that at first meditation will make you feel a lot like sitting around and doing nothing. However, the benefits of meditation will start showing up outside of your practice hours, so be certain to look for the changes meditation has brought to your life, outside of it. For instance, if you are able to focus more on listening to your partner, this may be the result of mindfulness meditation that will result in being more connected and intimate in your relationship.

According to Monahan, "One of the best ways to see those benefits is to get really clear on why you're meditating. If you can keep in mind what is motivating you (desire to be less stressed, to sleep better, to cultivate more self-love, etc.), you'll have an easier time staying committed to the practice and will more quickly notice when the benefits reveal themselves in your life outside of your practice."

When your practice mindfulness meditation regularly the benefits will affect both your mental and your physical health including managing depression, anxiety, relationship issues, sleep disorders, eating disorders, and stress. Your goal should be to make mindfulness meditation a regular occurrence in your daily life but if you have no time practicing every day you should not feel bad about it. There are various studies that support the fact that meditating four times per week can still offer you great benefits and by meditating regularly for eight weeks can actually alter the brain as discovered by neuroimaging studies. There is no reason for you to miss out on being healthier and leading a more stress-free and calm life.

AFTERWORD

Throughout the course of this book, we have covered a lot of ground about matters that are all connected to each other and will help you grow both in the physical and in the spiritual world. When it comes to your Third Eye, unlocking your sixth sense will open many doors through which you will gain wisdom and new experiences that will certainly help you grow in the physical world too. Many people have already opened their sixth sense without even realizing it and most ignore it altogether. Some others are totally afraid of the effects mostly because they do not practice controlling this enhanced sense.

The same principle applies to psychic abilities and with developing your connection with the astral plane as well as with protecting your aura. In the physical world, we are able to protect ourselves to some extent and the same should apply to our spirituality. Practicing healing meditation is one prevalent way, along with the others we have listed in this book, to protect your spiritual powers. As is the case with martial arts or any other skill we wish to develop, you should not stop practicing meditation and other methods such as affirmations, dream conversion, visualization, or hypnosis because they will help you protect, heal, cleanse, and nurture, your Third Eye chakra, your connection with the astral plane, your psychic abilities, your inner channels, and your aura.

Our mind is a tool that creates mental stories for us to help us navigate the world. It offers us maps. These maps are accessed through the Third Eye and by your developed psychic abilities. When you do not listen to your senses and what the universe tries to tell you, you will be at a loss when facing many difficulties in life. Even though we learn from our mistakes, the universe is here to help us and give us access to its endless knowledge. There is no reason for us to deny this kindness and ignore it as if it is nothing special.

People dedicate their whole lives to achieve such powers but not all of us can do this. Life can get in the way, but this is no reason to give up altogether. We can learn many things from people who spend their lives connecting with the universe and become the better version of ourselves by spending a few minutes each day to practice and develop our spiritual skills the same way we dedicate years of our lives to learn a set of skills that will help us navigate the physical world. We are all made up of energy and for this reason, do not make the mistake of ignoring our roots, where we came from, because our soul is eternal and is not limited by our physical bodies.